DIET

666

DEATH-DEFYING RESULTS

DIET 666

By Walter Labetti

Diet666.com

PREFACE

The time has finally come where I can honestly say beyond a doubt that I have a diet program that works very well. This came about after many years of trying different ways to lose weight with little or no success. There was some weight lost then I gained it right back even quicker than I lost it. These diets were like a roller-coaster ride, losing, losing, losing, then of course gaining, gaining, gaining— what a viscous cycle. Whether it was the high-protein diets or the minimum-calorie diets, they all failed. I tried eating one, two, three, four, or five meals a day, sometimes none. Sometimes I worked out at the gym losing 1,000 calories then ate 5,000 calories, which doesn't work! After doing intensive research and trying many different diets, I finally put everything together in a way that worked. I believe I have a complete weight loss program that is absolutely beyond a doubt much better than any other diet out there. I came up with Diet666, a success plan to say the least. If you have the determination, I have the plan.

Table of Contents

INTRODUCTION

This diet program, Diet666, was created after thoughtful considerations. Diet666 consists of a few components that when used correctly is a complete diet program that will produce amazing results. Diet666 is a complete diet program that works by each aspect of it contributing a significant component, and they all work together. When using this book, be determined to stick to all of the concepts as much as possible.

The primary components are eating six meals a day, doing six activities a day, and to do this for six days a week, followed by a day of fasting. Each aspect of Diet666 will be explained in detail as you read this book. There will be choices to be made concerning your goals, meals, activities, schedules, and fasting. I always found the hardest part of any diet was controlling hunger. By following the concepts of Diet666, it will not only help you lose weight, it will also curb your appetite. When Diet666 is performed over a long period of time it will lead you to achieving your goal weight. You will also be healthy and physically fit. There are numerous other benefits that can be very rewarding.

First, read the whole book then use it as a reference when needed. Create your own Diet666 program based on the concepts described in this book. Before implementing your personal Diet666 program, insure that you are healthy and ready to proceed. Configure your program at a level of intensity that's practical for your physical and mental abilities. In this book I will try my best to guide you along the journey of weight loss. It's an amazing feeling when you step onto that scale and notice how much weight you lost. Read the book, be determined, and treasure the results. Thanks for your interest in this unique Diet666 concept.

Chapter One

The Plan: six meals, six activities, six days a week, fast.

The plan works best when all the aspects of it are properly initiated. Try your best to adhere to all of the Diet666 concepts. Eating the six meals that are high in protein over the course of the day helps to keep your hunger at bay, but this alone is not enough to succeed. Performing six activities a day in conjunction with the six high-protein meals is the key to success. Activities can be much more than just fat-burning exercises. There are activities that are primarily used for burning calories while keeping you away from food. There are other activities that are less physical but keep your mind focused with no thoughts of food.

Following the Diet666 program with the six meals and six activities a day for six days a week and fasting becomes a way of life. By losing weight every single day, your body and mind accept this without a struggle. The seventh day is the day of fasting. There are no meals and there will only be consumption of non-calorie drinks. There will only be non-strenuous activities, unless of course you are performing at the Extreme666 level. The benefits of the day of fasting are losing weight, the body being relaxed, and the mind being focused. There are many other possible benefits to consider while fasting. Weighing yourself takes place on the day after the fast, only once a week. Eventually the level of neutrality is reached. This is when you reach your goal weight, and by having the set number of calories and activities on a daily basis, your weight is stabilized.

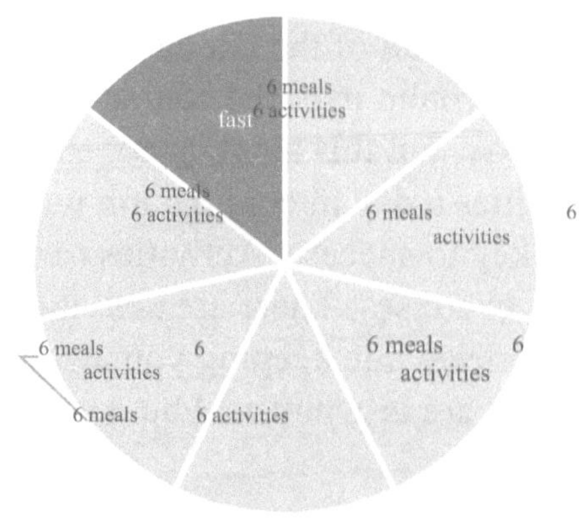

Good Habits, Bad Habits

When dealing with food, we all have habits—some good, and then
there are the bad ones. What I mean by a habit is a constant
occurrence, not the once in a while thing. There are some bad habits
that must be avoided. The number one thing to avoid is sugar. If you
are accustomed to massive amounts of sugar every day, it's best to
gradually get yourself off of the sugar fix. View sugar as a drug, it
can be addicting. Having excessive amounts is detrimental to
Diet666 and your health in general. Avoid all types of sugar! Get out
of the habit of adding sugar to anything, whether it's coffee, tea, or
while preparing food.

A common bad habit is eating meals that have a high calorie content
and are loaded with fat and sugar. A meal plan with one or two
meals a day is another bad habit. How about losing a few pounds

then gaining it right back? What about going out for dinner or going to a party and being compelled to eat a seven-course dinner? Whatever your bad habits may be, have resolve they will be recognized, understood, and overcome. When eating the proper six meals with high protein, no sugar, low carbohydrates, and low fats, there is a path to success.

The six meals a day will keep you nourished and over time, it will be one of the best habits you ever developed. Performing the six activities a day with their many benefits will be something that you look forward to, and this also will be a great habit you've gotten into. By doing this for six days a week, it will strengthen you physically and, most of all, mentally. Day after day, week after week, over and over, this diet plan will not only be a great habit you adapted to, it will also be the way you naturally live your life.

Determination and Mindset

When considering the reasons why a person would want to lose weight, there are many. These reasons are different for each of us. It seems to me the top reasons for losing weight are to look good and be healthy, in that order. When being at the proper weight, things are easier, like getting into a pair of pants or walking up a flight of stairs. Examine and consider your abilities, goals, wishes, and dreams.

By using this book, you will configure a solid weight loss program to accomplish your goals. There are the small segments within Diet666 that consist of consuming meals and performing activities, these will be your mini accomplishments. These accomplishments over time will lead to major results, long-term weight loss, and ultimately reaching your goal weight.

The process starts by knowing your abilities and having a powerful determination. Decide on what your schedule will be for your six meals, six activities, six days a week and fasting. Know what your choice of meals and activities will be. Keep focused on the ultimate goal, it's to lose weight, be healthy, and have a sound mind. Do not let anyone or anything sidetrack you. If you make Diet666 the most important thing in your life, and in fact it may be, you will surely succeed.

Avoid the foods that will impair your diet. Avoid the people, places, and situations that will lead you toward overeating or not doing your activities. Know your personality. Are you the type of person that easily gives up on things? If you are in this category, start slowly by gradually decreasing your daily calorie intake. Slowly increase the duration and difficulty of your activities. Choose mini fasts at first and then gradually increase their duration as the weeks go on.

Diet666 has limitless options. Create the plan that suits yourself. If you have that extreme type of personality, go for it! Ensure that you are mentally and physically fit. You can always adjust the plan as needed. Put yourself ahead of all other things in life. Embrace activities that will keep you safely away from overeating. Activities will also be used to burn fat, whether in little portions or by massive amounts.

Yes, there will be bumps in the road like most things in life, that's just how life is. Always look forward to getting on the scale, the once a week pleasure that lets you know it is so much worth the everyday dedication in which you conduct yourself. Know that there are people that try but never do, you are the one that tries very hard and succeeds. Know the longer you are into this Diet666 plan, the easier it gets. Your hunger will be diminished, your fat will melt away, and the unhealthy style of overeating will be a thing of the distant past. This book, along with your unsurpassed determination, will undoubtedly produce the results you're entitled to.

Past Failures

When people tell me about their failed weight loss attempts, a few things are heard over and over. The one that I never accept is the line "I just can't do it." Unless the person is physically or mentally incapable, yes, they can. Of course, they can. It just means to me that the method they're using is not a complete diet plan, or maybe it's too hard, not understood, too complicated, or they lack determination.

There are those that say, "I follow my diet but can't lose weight." This is usually from those diet plans that are not a functional, systematic weight loss program. I know there are people who can eat all day long and they won't gain any weight whatsoever. For most of us, the "eat as much as you want whenever you want" types of diets equal disaster. Have a look at your past failed attempts to lose weight and examine the reasons.

For me, what has always done me in was that the hunger would overcome my willpower. I got weak and the diet went out the window. I told myself lies, like, "I will only eat half of the hero," "I'm at the movies so it's okay to eat a large popcorn," or "It's my birthday, so it's alright to eat 4,000 calories." I took a close look at the previous diet plans I tried to no avail. I discovered that there were a few commonalities. These diets were limited in structure and had poor weight lose concepts. When using these types of methods, I would constantly be hungry, lose my determination, then finally give up altogether. It took me many failed attempts to finally devise a plan that works well without a crazy amount of effort. Diet666 is where it's at!

Please folks, if this is your tenth broken scale in two weeks, it wasn't the scale's fault you didn't lose weight! Do not let past failures stop you from creating a better you. Having tried is a lot better than never giving it a try at all. Yes, it may not have worked for a variety of reasons. There are positive things that took place, you wanted change, you followed a path toward losing weight, and you gave it some level of effort.

As you read this book, you will have better insight as to why you didn't have the success with the other diet plans. That was the past, now's the time to follow Diet666 with confidence and determination. My intention is not to criticize other diet plans, I'm just trying to explain why Diet666 is the best. Please don't consider losing less than expected weight as a failure, it's not! We all lose weight at different rates. Adjust if necessary but don't quit. Know that having an appetite, being a little hungry, or very hungry, is normal and controllable.

Why This Over Others?

Diet666 is designed for the primary reason of losing weight. Yes, there are other benefits that you will see along the way. I don't suggest this diet is beneficial in curing or helping any illness, disorder, or disease, but it may. This diet is new, and the research needs to be done before I would make any such claims.

There are thousands of diet plans out there with all different strategies and promises. Some of the most popular diet plans are only concerned with your daily calorie content. We all heard of diets where only eating one type of food group will work miracles. Diet plans of only eating fish, meat, poultry, vegetables, cheese burgers, etc. There are mail order food supply diets based on the theory that if you only eat their products, you will be guaranteed to lose weight. There are diets that claim you can eat as much as you want as long as you burn off the calories. Sounds good, but are they? There are diets that claim you can easily lose weight by only being concerned with burning calories and nothing else. There are the quick fixes with a variety of medical procedures, tummy tucks or gastral bypasses to mention a few. There are a variety of weight loss pills. Some weight loss pills are available over-the-counter with no proven results and others that are FDA approved.

Consider the effort it takes to lose 1,000 calories and how easy it is to consume 1,000 calories. For the vast majority of us, it is much easier to gain weight than it is to lose weight. This is why it takes a comprehensive weight loss program (Diet666) to lose weight and keep it off. Quick fixes work for a short time and some don't work at all. Diet666 surely is concerned with calorie counts, but only counting calories leads to failure. Activities alone are important, but by themselves will fail. The same holds true for the hundreds of fad diets. Diet666 is a complete package with all the necessary components that work together to produce amazing results.

Now, I will give you some detail why this works better than any other diet, then in further chapters the diet will be fully explained.

The six-meal system is calorie and nutritionally controlled. The meals are high in protein while being low in carbohydrates, low in fat, and no sugar. This is a major part in keeping you with little or no hunger between meals and maintaining your muscle mass.

The six activities a day will keep you focused on what you are doing and not on food. This works in conjunction with the six-meal system. If possible, one of the six activities should be a physical, fat burning exercise. Choosing your activities will depend on the intensity of your chosen plan. The activities that are more intense will build muscle, burn calories, and also be fun.

The next aspect is doing this for six days a week, which helps to make the whole diet a good habit. The body will adjust to burning stored body fat.

The seventh day is the day of fasting. This does a few things. It relaxes and cleanses your body of salt and toxins while focusing and strengthening your mind. There will also be a significant number of calories lost.

An added benefit of Diet666 is that it gets easier the longer it's followed. Burning fat every day will be the way your body naturally functions. As a whole, from my personal experiences, this diet by far surpasses all the others by leaps and bounds. I don't claim to be an expert nutritionist or dietician. I'm not a sports trainer or professional athlete. I am the one who created Diet666; I used it and I know it works.

Diet666 vs. High-Protein Diets

These high-protein diets are the types of diets that primarily focus on consuming meals that are high in protein and little else. These types of dieting programs are incomplete, but with some changes can be incorporated into our Diet666 plan.

These high-protein diets fall short by not properly planning for your entire day or weeks. Diet666 does far more than only focusing on high-protein meals. With Diet666, it's six high-protein meals, six times a day, for six days a week, then a day of fasting. Very important aspects of Diet666 are the six activities a day, six days a week. The day of fasting is another important part of the full Diet666 concept. Diet666 is a complete plan, which by far surpasses the limited high-protein diets. Diet666, by including high-protein meals along with activities and fasting, makes it more of a lifelong plan, not just a quick fix for a short time.

Diet666 vs. Low-Carbohydrate Diets

These types of diets that only focus on consuming a restricted amount of carbohydrates fall short at being a complete long-term diet. Consuming low carbohydrates is a good starting point, and making adjustments can be incorporated into the Diet666 program. Diet666 does far more than only focusing on low-carbohydrate meals. With the Diet666 program, it's six high-protein meals, six times a day, for six days a week. Very important aspects of Diet666 are the six activities a day throughout six days a week. The day of fasting is another important part of the full Diet666 concept. Diet666 is a complete plan, which by far surpasses the limited low-carbohydrate diets. Diet666, by including six high-protein meals along with six activities and fasting makes it more of a complete plan, not just a fad diet.

Diet666 vs. Pre-Packaged Meal Diet

There are various diet plans that are based on preparing, packaging, and delivering their meals for your convenience. Each of these plans have their own types of meals with different proportions of nutrients. These plans have the convenience of having a delivery system, but there is a significant monetary price to pay. Diet666 has much more to offer; it's a compressive all-inclusive diet plan. With its six meals, six activities, and fasting, losing weight will be achieved and maintained.

Diet666 vs. Diets Based on Selling Their Various Products

There are diet plans that sell products to support your nutrition, supplement your vitamin and mineral requirements, along with appetite suppressants. These diet plans may include various drinks for nutrition and diet bars for snacks. These diet plans are lacking in structure. Diet plans like these may be beneficial for a few days, but they don't have what it takes to be a solid, effective plan for a longer duration. Diet666 is a comprehensive diet plan that will consistently produce results for days, weeks, months, or years, with no gimmicks involved.

Diet666 vs. Diet Plans Working on a Point System

These types of diet programs work on a point system. There are different types of foods that have a different point value. By maintaining the proper amount of points, supposedly weight will be lost. For these types of weight loss programs there typically are support centers. Where these weight loss programs fall short is that they are deficient in activities. They don't have a plan of how to use your time productively. Diet666, in addition to eating high-protein meals, has the benefit of the activities and fasting.

Diet666 vs. Various Mediterranean/European Diets

The typical concept of these types of diets is to consume large amounts of healthy fats, such as olive oil. These diets also include fish, poultry, vegetables, fruits, cheese, nuts, grains, legumes, and yogurt. These diets have an emphasis on having low amounts of red meat and sugar. These diets, when performed correctly, may be healthy, but for losing weight they are not the optimum choice. Diet666 is a multifaceted weight loss program, which focuses on high-protein meals along with activities and fasting. This makes it a much better choice for losing and maintaining your weight loss.

Diet666 vs. Vegan and Vegetarian Diets

These are the diets that restrict animal products to various extents. Most vegan diets totally eliminate all animal products. There are many types of vegetarian diets, each with its own limitations on animal products.

Most of these types of diets totally eliminate the consumption of meat, fish, and poultry. These diets can be healthy, while being morally and spiritually rewarding, but they're not the premium weight loss program. These diet concepts can be integrated into Diet666. Adjusting to six high-protein meals, and adding the six activities and fasting, will make this a vegan/vegetarian Diet666 program. For a vegan to get complete proteins and restrict their calorie intake at the same time can be challenging, but it surely is possible.

Diet666 vs. Fasting Diets

There are many variations of fasting diets that are used for different reasons, whether spiritual, to control an illness, or weight loss, to name a few. Controlling weight loss by fasting alone would be an incomplete program and can also be dangerous. Fasting for many consecutive days with total food deprivation can bring a person toward malnutrition with the possibility of many other health issues. There are fasting diets that can last for any number of days. There are fasts that restrict a variety of foods and even liquids.

Diet666 uses a fast one day per week, which I consider useful but not dangerous. Diet666 is a multifaceted weight loss program that can be adjusted for your personal preferences and will produce the needed results for as long as you desire. You'll be rewarded in many ways, not just your amazing weight loss.

Diet666 vs. Calorie-Counting Diets

The calorie-counting diets are good in a sense that they restrict calories to help you lose weight, but without controlling the proper nutritional contents this can be disastrous. When using these diets, even if the proper nutrition was controlled, they would still be lacking in the necessary components that are required for a complete diet program.

Diet666 uses calorie counting at an advanced level in conjunction with the six meals, six activities, and fasting concept. Diet666 is a complete diet program.

Preparing for Obstacles

There most certainly will be obstacles, but most of them can be overcome with the simple methods described in this book. Get professional medical assistance if you have a mental or physical impairment. Consult with a medical doctor if there is any inkling that it might be needed, the priority is to be healthy and safe at all times. Getting the approval of a medical doctor is the safe way to go.

Being very overweight won't be an obstacle if handled the right way and under the supervision of a professional medical doctor. If this is the case, start your Diet666 program at a very easy level. Start with the same number of calories you are accustomed to and spread them out over the six meals a day. Perform the six activities a day limiting them to ones with little or no exertion. You can gradually decrease the calories and increase the intensity of the activities with the supervision of a medical doctor if needed.

Obstacles can be getting fatigued, exhausted, or overly hungry. Always stay hydrated by drinking plenty of non-calorie liquids such as water. Drink limited amounts of caffeinated drinks, which can lead to dehydration and insomnia. During workouts if you are feeling overly tired, have a drink, slow down, or stop altogether. Have a meal, take a rest, lay down, or take a nap. Switch to a non-intensive, relaxing activity.

The hunger factor can wreak havoc on the diet if not handled properly. By strictly following this diet you can bring this problem down to a minimum. Hunger comes on slowly; notice it and control it. At the first sign of hunger, have a drink; perform an activity, the physical or focused ones work best; have one of the six meals; take a shower; go for a swim; have a cup of coffee; go for a walk out of the house; get far away from food; take a nap; or go to sleep. There are options, handling it at the onset is best. There are times when you feel hungry but it's really dehydration, fatigue, stress, or a lack of sleep. Our bodies and minds sometimes misinterpret these feelings.

What do you do when you're sitting at a table with lots of food, either at a restaurant, a barbeque, or a party? Sip sparkling water, not wine or beer. If the duration is long, have one of your meals every hour or so. Eat small portions of protein and vegetables as your dinner servings. Incorporate your activities in-between the meals. Socialize, walk, dance, find something to do, be active.

If you have a cold or perhaps the flu, take your medication, rest, have your six meals, and do six light activities like reading a book.

Prioritizing

We can make the decision of what is more important, losing weight or eating in excess? What are we willing to give up in order to have a better body, a more productive life, and probably live a little longer? The answer isn't so simple, it's a bit more than to just limit your calorie intake. What's your food of choice? Chocolate, ice cream, pizza, burgers, etc.? There's also the other high calorie, high carbohydrate stuff like beer, wine, and alcohol. Besides doing away with the bad stuff, it's the work of introducing the good meals and activities into your life that make an impact. There is the discipline of restructuring your life with the priority on losing weight. After thoroughly reading this book, make the decision on what level of weight loss you can handle. What are you willing to give up or limit? What are the activities you will perform and what can't you do without? Honestly, find your priority and be true to yourself when customizing your plan.

Purpose of Food, Pleasure, and Effects

We live in a food-on-demand society with numerous foods just minutes away. Humans are nourished on a daily basis even though we are designed to go days without food. What we consume directly affects our health.

When eating the proper foods in the right portions, we will lose weight and be healthy at the same time. There are affects from eating certain foods that may go unnoticed. The affects will be clear once the plan is implemented.

On a daily basis we must stay hydrated by drinking plenty of water. The need for eating complete proteins is also a major priority. Protein keeps hunger away along with building muscle.

Pure sugar and high sugar items must be totally eliminated. Sugar adds unnecessary calories and is unhealthy. Sugar has an added consequence, it makes you hungry. NO SUGAR! Other food groups are necessary but minimize the complex carbohydrates and fats. Most vegetables are good but stay away from high sugar fruits. It's good to take a daily multivitamin and have fiber in your diet. Use other nutritional supplements as needed.

Eating because of boredom or for recreation is quite common, but it is a habit to be avoided. Instead, perform an activity, keep busy, or go for a walk, but don't use food as a recreation. The social aspect of enjoying food with other people is a culture we're accustomed to. The secret is being prepared and to work this into your overall plan.

Want something fun to do? Let's go out for dinner, have some snacks, or maybe ice cream! Sound familiar? There're other ways to have fun. Don't use food as a recreational tool, you'll be sorry later. It's no fun putting on the unwanted weight. Get accustomed to using food for a purpose. Something that is going to benefit you in a specific way. Don't reward yourself by overeating, use a different method. Know the results of everything you eat and drink. Treat sugar as a deadly drug. For some people it truly is. Know when you eat a little sugar, you want more. When coming down from the sugar high you will be very hungry.

Read This Book, Evaluate, Adjust

Thoroughly read and understand this book. Take notes when necessary. Regard this book as your bible toward losing weight. The plan is quite simple and straightforward. When broken down into individual segments, it can get quite complex. The better you understand the underlying interactions with meals, activities, and fasting, the easier it will be to create and implement the plan.

As you're proceeding with this diet plan, use the book as a reference guide. From time to time reevaluate how it's going and what could better suit yourself. Readjust your plan as necessary but try not to do this every day. If possible, make your adjustments at the beginning of the following week. You may want to increase or decrease your daily calorie count. You may want to adjust your activities to more or less strenuous. You may want to introduce or do away with some activities. You may find it better to fast on a different day, one that is more convenient. As your life changes, the time sequences of meals, activities, and fasting might need modifications. This plan is very versatile, there's an endless amount of options.

Simple or Intricate?

There are many ways to configure your personal Diet666 plan. One way is you can simply have the same types of meals over and over again and use the same set of activities every day, that's perfectly fine. You can make gourmet meals if that's what you prefer. If you're a vegan, vegetarian, or need other specialty food, that's fine also. Perhaps it's sushi you prefer, that's absolutely doable. Stay within your calorie count and be mindful of the diet's nutritional structure.

Your activities can be a short walk six times a day with little exertion. There are many other non-strenuous activities that can be used, like reading, writing, etc. More vigorous activities can be accomplished like weight training, body building, or perhaps developing your favorite sport. The regiment of six activities a day still applies.

The day of fasting can be simply drinking water and meditating all day. You can diversify the day with flavored non-calorie drinks, sparkling water, tea, or coffee. There are a lot of non-calorie drinks to choose from. You can see your favorite movie, do some yoga, or listen to music. Add things that make your day exciting.

Why It Gets Easier

It gets easier as the days go on because your body gets accustomed to having meals high in protein six times a day. Your mind gets in sync with the activities and meals. Consuming six meals a day with six activities a day and doing so six days a week will make this plan habit-forming. As you become regimental, the process of fasting becomes quite easy.

After performing this diet for a length of time, your body gets accustomed to burning your body fat and using it for energy. Our bodies are well prepared for this. Our ancestors were accustomed to this process, but with modern food sources, we are not. When we are deficient in calories, we burn body fat for energy. When we have excess calories, our body stores it as fat. It really is an amazing process.

Up until this point your body was probably not used to burning body fat. If you were eating excess calorie amounts, your body became very good at storing it as body fat. Now it's time to reverse the process, burn the fat, use it for energy, and lose the weight. Seeing the extra weight fading away will definitely keep you motivated. Getting into the next size down pants is a great morale booster.

Where to Start?

This is the simplified version that you will build on. The first thing that needs to be done is for you to read and fully understand the entire book. Take notes. Go over the book a few times if needed. Devise the right plan for yourself using the concepts described in this book. Determine what your meals will be, what the calorie amounts for each meal will be, and at what times you will have them. Determine what your activities will be, their durations, and when to use them. It's best to have an activity planned between the meals.

Throughout the day, it will be a meal then an activity with some time in-between each. You will be doing these six meals and six activities every day for six days. Plan the time you want to wake up and go to sleep during the day of fasting. Plan what liquids you will drink and what activities you will do, if any. Get a medical checkup from a qualified medical doctor. Explain your plan to your doctor and what your intentions are, ensuring it's safe for you to proceed. The diet will be more detailed in further chapters.

The Rewards

We all have our special reasons for losing weight. I'm sure yours are good! One thing for sure is that there's nothing like achieving your goal, especially when it makes a better you. So, what are the rewards besides cherishing your achievement? For one thing, you probably will live a bit longer, but that pales in comparison to just looking great.

When you lose weight, it seems like life just opens up for you. All physical things are easier, and you feel better about yourself. You're ready to take on the world. People look at you a little different or better. Slipping into those once tight jeans is an accomplishment in itself. Being proud of yourself makes it so much easier to carry on in life and with your Diet666.

Level of Neutrality

Here is my fundamental theory of neutrality. I'm sure it's not a unique theory but it's worth mentioning nonetheless. A person's body weight is dependent on his/her caloric intake. I believe that if there is a group of people of various weights having the same metabolic rate and other equivalent contributing factors, such as energy usage and consuming the same number of calories each day, their weights will converge and remain stable given the necessary time.

Using the rough concept that for every pound of weight that a person weighs there needs to be ten calories to sustain it. This means that whatever someone's starting weight is, if they constantly consumed 1,500 calories a day, they would eventually reach the weight of 150 lbs. That's right, whether a person is 300 lbs. or 100 lbs. when starting, by consuming 1,500 calories every day, they will arrive at 150 lbs.

This theory is good to know because it shows you one of the underlying processes of weight control. You will reach your target weight then you will maintain that weight by using the concepts set forth in Diet666.

Chapter Two
Six Meals a Day

Why Six?

Six meals with the right nutritional content will keep your body sustained over the course of the day. The meals will give you the protein necessary to keep your hunger at a low level and under control. The protein also helps to prevent your body from burning muscle for energy. This six-meal system is a lot different than the traditional three meals per day, which most of us are accustomed to. The three-meal system is more conducive toward gaining weight, not losing weight. With only three meals, it's easy for your appetite to increase to a point where it's out of control. As you limit the calories and provide high proportions of protein in each of the six meals, your body will become very efficient at burning off the stored body fat. Your body will be burning fat off all day and every day, reducing hunger and losing weight. The full effects of this will be apparent after a few weeks.

Meal Contents and Nutrition

The individual meals are primarily based on complete proteins. In the area of eighty percent protein, ten percent fat, ten percent complex carbohydrates, and zero sugar. The overall total daily nutrition intake should have some vegetables, fiber, fat, and complex carbohydrates. Daily multivitamins are recommended. Use supplements as needed to get your total nutritional requirements. As you go forward you will get better at adding fiber, vegetables, vitamins, and minerals to your meals.

There are a lot of creative ways to get complete proteins. Fish, poultry, meat, and dairy products are the most popular complete proteins. Every meal doesn't need to be complete in all the necessary proteins, but every meal with complete proteins is best. When I mention complete proteins, I mean the necessary combination of amino acids that you need to consume on a daily basis. The next best thing to having complete proteins is to have incomplete proteins that don't have all the necessary amino acids. Through the day, these incomplete proteins will interact with your complete high-protein meals.

Incomplete proteins are things like grains, seeds, nuts, and legumes that are consumed separately. By preparing meals with a combination of grains, seeds, nuts, and legumes, complete protein meals will be achieved. If it's going to be a non-protein meal, which I don't recommend, it should be based on vegetables and/or complex carbohydrates, not sugars or high fat.

There are many different combinations of foods that will be used for your meals. Have many varieties of food available that you'll be using and focus on quality protein. Avoid having readily available sugary or high carbohydrates products. You will get Diet666 down to a science by doing so in your own specific way. It will be your overall plan, your meals, activities, fasting, weight loss, and ultimately your personal accomplishments.

Foods to Use, Foods to Avoid

The one food source to totally eliminate is any type of pure sugar. I don't mean the small amounts you will get from vegetables or fruit. I mean refined cane sugar, brown sugar, unrefined sugar, honey, etc. The products with high sugar content should be avoided at all costs, such as candy, ice cream, cakes, cookies, pies, pastries, etc. Fruits high in sugar content should be avoided, such as oranges, grapes, cherries, etc. Remember, the sugar will enhance your appetite and make you very hungry.

Avoid high carbohydrate foods, such as white flower bread, pasta, potatoes, white rice, beer, wine, alcohol, etc. Avoid high fat content foods, such as cheese, bacon, fried foods, salad dressings, cheese sauces, processed meats, etc. Fats are very high in calorie content and some are unhealthy. Olive oil is the better choice in the fat group.

Some carbohydrates and fats are needed in our daily nutrition but only in small amounts. If eating bread or flour-based products, use whole wheat or multi-grain. Choose the low calorie, high fiber bread.

When using meat use lean cuts. Beef cuts that are lean are the eye round, top round, and bottom round. For poultry, select turkey or chicken breast, without the skin and not cooked in fat. Most types of fish are high in protein and low in fat. Complete proteins can be achieved with combinations of legumes and whole grains. Soy and tofu are good sources of complete proteins. If using protein bars, choose the ones with no or low sugar, low carbohydrates, and low in fat.

How Food Works on the Body

The first step of food acting on your body takes place on the mind long before eating. Think about this for a while, this must be remembered, it will save you from going down the wrong path. Billions of dollars are spent in advertisement specifically designed to have you consume unhealthy food. The sight, smell, sounds, or thoughts of food are the first interaction with your body. The advertisements appear on television, on storefronts, billboards, cellphones, or the radio. The influence is all around us. We have many great associations with food that trigger hunger. Don't fall into that trap.

Keep in mind that sleeplessness, tiredness, and dehydration can also make you feel hungry. The next step toward eating is our mind choosing to eat and what to eat. It's not often that we think about why we are eating. "Why are we eating?" should be the first thought. By starting with "why," a logical decision can be made.

The priority in choosing food should be of nutritional value. Try your hardest to eat for purpose not for fun. The fun is losing weight, being healthy, and looking great.

Now for some of the interactions that food will have on our body. Water is used throughout the body for all of its functions. Protein builds and repairs body tissue, bone, skin, muscle, and blood. The body can also use protein for energy or change it into fat and store it.

Protein in our body consists of basically twenty amino acids, and out of the twenty, there are nine that are essential. The nine essential amino acids cannot be made by our bodies, so they must be obtained on a daily basis. Most diets will recommend having complete proteins three times a day. This diet plan recommends that the essential nine amino acids be consumed six times a day.

Carbohydrates, simple or complex, are needed in the body on a daily basis in small amounts. Some people think carbohydrates are not needed at all. Do not consume simple carbohydrates, which are basically pure sugar. Do not consume products with a moderate amount of sugar. Refined sugar quickly goes into the blood giving you energy, and then it exits, leaving you with a feeling of hunger and other ill effects. An overabundance of sugar will be stored as fat. Complex carbohydrates go into the blood at a slower rate, providing sustained energy with less of a hunger sensation afterwards.

Use complex carbohydrates sparingly, because some have large amounts of calories. An overabundance of complex carbohydrates will be stored as fat. Complex carbohydrates contain fiber, vitamins, and various amounts of sugar. It's best to get complex carbohydrates from whole grains, legumes, or vegetables. Avoid high sugar fruits.

Fats are necessary for the body functions and can also provide energy. When there is a surplus of fat in the body, it is stored. When it is necessary, the stored fat will be used for energy. Unhealthy fats are basically derived from animals, poultry, and dairy products. Some more healthy sources of fats are from corn, olives, nuts, seeds, avocado, palm, soy, and coconut. I tend to use extra virgin olive oil.

There are many indirect sources of fat, the ones you may not know about. There are many products that contain fat and may taste good, but they are loaded with calories. The most notable products are the ones that are baked or fried. Fats are packed with calories, so use only healthy ones and use them sparingly. Some healthy fats come from fish like salmon, mackerel, sardines, and trout. Other healthy fats come from olive, walnut, canola, and safflower oil.

Vitamins and minerals are necessary for the body to function properly. It can be difficult to get all the necessary vitamins and minerals on a daily basis. I recommend a multivitamin and mineral supplement if needed. Use other supplements as needed. I suggest you do further reading on the subject of nutrition. It will be helpful, interesting, and may be one of your six activities!

The Meal Schedules

When preparing for your meal schedule, there are a few things to consider. Consider the times of your meals in conjunction with the activities you will be doing. Think about your everyday personal events, whether it's work or your other responsibilities. Plan on how the meals will be paced within your overall every day Diet666 structure. Think about the places where each meal will be consumed.

Also, consider the time you wake up and the time you go to sleep. Calculate the time frame of your awake hours. If you're sleeping eight hours, the awake hours are sixteen. Try to even out the meals with activities between them. It may be that you wake up around eight a.m. then wait a while, maybe a few hours, before you have your first meal. You will then have one of your six meals at every two hours.

In between your meals you will be doing one of your six daily activities. A total of six meals and six activities daily for six days. On the seventh day is the fast. This is the basic concept of the meal schedule, but it doesn't need to have the exact meal contents, number of calories, or time sequences.

Preparing Daily and Weekly Meals

After devising the schedule of your choice, it's time to choose the meal content. There should be an emphasis on high-protein meals. There should be no pure sugar in the meals. Through the course of the day you should have little complex carbohydrates and fats. There are many types of food products to choose from. Determine what's needed for the week based on your planned calorie levels and nutritional content.

Don't forget the liquids, whether it is water or other drinks. Liquids are basically to keep you hydrated. Liquids high in protein, low in carbohydrates, and low in fats can also be consumed as a meal.

Multivitamins should also be on your shopping list. Everyone's personally designed meal plans will differ, you must choose what additional supplements are needed. For instance, if there's no calcium in your diet plan, take a calcium supplement. The emphasis for every meal will be on high protein, low fat, and low carbohydrates.

Choosing your daily calorie count can differ in a few ways. One way is to start with your normal every day calorie count, that is the number of calories consumed before starting Diet666. Divide that number of calories by six. Six, meaning six meals. If you previously consumed 2,400 calories daily, you will now have six meals of 400 calories each. After a day or so, systemically decrease the calories at your own pace until you reach a point where you're losing weight.

To show you a different way, first choose the total amount of calories you will have for the day then divide that by six. For example, prepare six meals for the first day. Six sandwiches each consisting of one slice of low-calorie whole-wheat bread, three ounces of deli sliced turkey breast, and a few pieces of lettuce. This would be a total of about 1,020 calories for the day. Each of the six meals would be approximately 170 calories. After a day or so, you could diminish the turkey content of each meal by one-half ounce until you reach your goal calorie content. You could use many variations to achieve the same results.

There could be different meals throughout the day to achieve your daily calorie count, then as the days go on have fewer calories. The important thing is to have complete proteins six times, paced throughout the day.

Your goal is to get to the point where you always consume less calories than what your body needs on a daily basis. This is the training process of getting your body to burn its stored fat and use it for energy. It takes a while, but when your body is fully accustomed to this, losing weight takes little effort.

Choose meals that are high in protein with some healthy fat and little complex carbohydrates. No sugar.

The following chart shows the ideal goal of nutritional proportions.

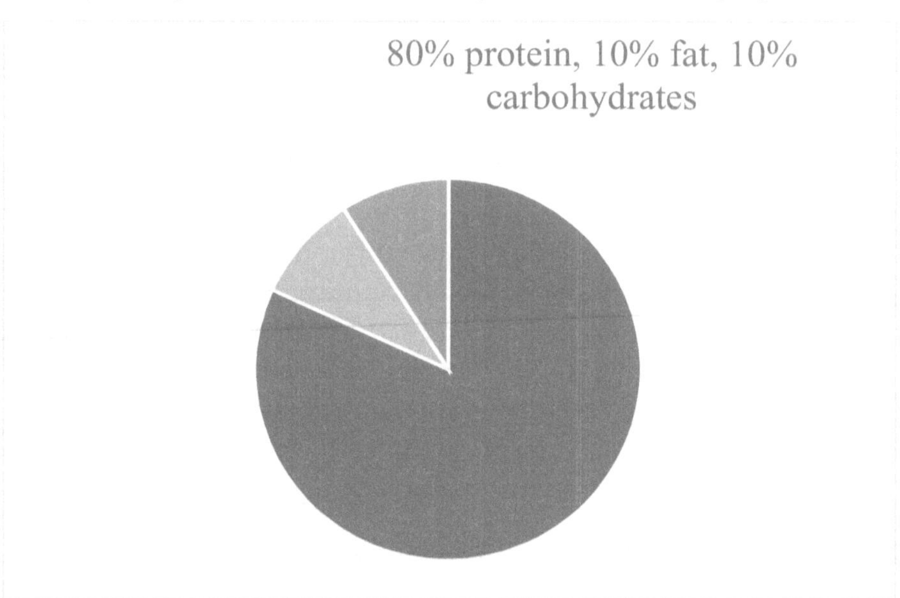

Liquids

Liquids come in many forms and contain many types of nutritional components. The main purpose of a liquid is to provide water for the body. Hydration is probably the most important thing to sustaining life. We need water throughout the day. Without an adequate supply of water, our bodily functions are impaired. Simply spoken, we can't function properly without an abundance of water. Some signs of dehydration are headache, fatigue, tiredness, and yes, hunger.

Throughout the day drink plenty of water or other liquids that don't contain sugar. This will include flavored water, sparkling water, or diet drinks. Tea and coffee are all right when used wisely. Caffeinated drinks can be a diuretic, they will unintentionally remove water from the body. Caffeinated drinks can subdue hunger, so use them in moderation as needed.

There are fortified drinks that are packed with protein. Unfortunately, a lot of these drinks carry unnecessary calories. When selecting these types of drinks for a meal get the ones that are high in protein and low in fat and low in carbohydrates.

Stay clear of all the drinks with huge amounts of sugar. The juice drinks sound healthy but usually are packed with sugar. The ice cream drinks are high in both fat and sugar. You can make your own nutritious drinks concentrating on high protein, no sugar, low carbohydrates, and low fats. Remember to keep in line with your calorie count.

When you're between meals and you start to feel hungry, have a water or other drink then continue with one of your activities. Remember, sometimes the mind will interpret dehydration for hunger.

On the day of fasting I suggest you have many different types of non-caloric drinks at hand. It's nice to have choices, especially considering that you'll just be having liquids all day.

Calorie Count

The simplified definition of a calorie is a unit of energy that food gives us when consumed. To memorize all the amounts of calories and nutritional value in every type of food would be difficult, if not impossible. The easy way to do this is to have a pocket calorie counter or a cellphone app that has the basic foods giving you their calorie amounts and nutritional values. The foods you commonly use will be memorized. After a while you'll be able to approximate most foods.

There are calorie-loaded foods that are of little good to us, like pure sugar and simple carbohydrates. There are foods with enormous amounts of calories that are sparingly needed, those are the fats. When it comes to complete protein foods, there are some that are low in calories but high in protein. It can be a challenge to get enough complete proteins without animal products.

When obtaining complete proteins by mixing grains with legumes, nuts, or seeds, we tend to have a disproportional number of calories from carbohydrates and fats vs. protein. It absolutely can be achieved; it's very important to know your calorie count and nutritional properties of your selected meals. You want the protein without the unnecessary calories.

A lot of food products now have the calories and nutritional values printed on the packaging. If you haven't done so yet, start reading the packaging on all the food you purchase, you'll get to know and understand food much better. There are things in the grocery store like vegetables and fruits that aren't packaged and don't have their nutritional values posted. This is where your calorie counter comes in handy, or you could access the internet to find the answer.

When you go out for dinner, most of the time there are no calorie or nutritional aspects posted. Hopefully by the time you finish this book you will have enough knowledge to survive your dining experience without going over your intended calorie count. You'll be able to make wise choices based on the knowledge you have.

After a few weeks or perhaps months, you'll always know the calories you consume and all the nutritional properties. You'll also know all the calories you are using through the day, that's calories consumed, calories used, and the calories you lost. There will be variations in the weekly losses due to changes in your meals, activities, water retention, and a changing metabolism.

Calorie Calculations

Knowing the calories entering and leaving the body is a must. First, let's estimate the calories needed to maintain your current weight. This will be the number of calories to sustain your current weight without considering any activities that will burn off calories. Keep in mind everyone has a different metabolism because we all burn calories at a different rate.

Here's how to estimate the needed calories to maintain your current weight. Multiply your current weight by ten. So, if your current weight is 200 lbs., you will need 2,000 calories to maintain this weight (200 X 10 = 2,000 calories). To lose one pound you must have a deficiency of 3,500 calories. When you are deficient in calories at the end of the day, you lose weight. By performing certain activities, you will burn calories. By following this Diet666 plan you will be doing both, consuming less than needed calories and also burning calories by performing activities.

To get an accurate reading on your weight loss when weighing yourself, it's best to wear the same clothing if any, every time. I recommend weighing yourself once a week the day after your fast, which is also the beginning of your new week.

The areas of weight loss on the body will vary from person to person, there are many areas where the body stores fat. It seems for me when losing weight, the last place to lose it is from my hips. What I have noticed during this diet is, I never lose the exact amount of weight which was calculated for the week. Sometimes it's drastically more or less, or off by a few pounds. The good news is over time it averages out. If you lose twelve pounds the first week then only a few pounds the next week, don't be surprised. In time you will lose as much as you desire.

Let's examine how it works as far as calories in and out. Keep in mind there's a lot more to this diet than just calories in and out. If your weight is 200 pounds, your daily sustainable calorie count is 2,000. If you decrease your calories by fifty percent and burn off one thousand calories a day for six days, this will be a loss of 12,000 calories. Add to that the day of fasting for another 2,000 calories. The total calorie loss is 14,000 calories. Divide the 14,000 calories by 3,500 (for one pound) and you have a loss of four pounds. That's just what I did for a few weeks.

You should have in addition to a calorie counter, a small food scale that will be useful in determining portion sizes. There's an abundance of information just by reading food labels, but that's not adequate. I will now give you some calorie counts as a starting point for your nutritional knowledge base. The following nutritional approximations will help you make wise choices.

Alfalfa sprouts, 1/2 cup, 40 calories, 1 gram of protein, 0 fat, 0 carbohydrates.
Apple-one medium size, 55 calories, 0 protein, 0 fat, 15 grams of carbohydrates.
Apricot-one medium size, 17 calories, 0 protein, 0 fat, 4 grams of carbohydrates.
Artichoke hearts, 1 oz., canned in water, 25 calories, 1gram of protein, 2 grams of fat, 5 grams of carbohydrates.
Bacon, 3 strips cooked, 109 calories, 6 grams of protein, 9 grams of fat, 0 carbohydrates.
Bacon/turkey, 1 strip, 25 calories, 2 grams of protein, 2 grams of fat, 0 carbohydrates.
Bagel-one medium, 289 calories, 11 grams of protein, 2 grams of fat, 56 grams of carbohydrates.
Banana-one medium, 121 calories, 1 gram of protein, 0 fat, 31 grams of carbohydrates.
Barbeque sauce, 2 tbsp., 52 calories, 0 protein, 0 fat, 13 grams of carbohydrates.
Barley-cooked, 6 oz., 190 calories, 4 grams of protein, 1 gram of fat, 44 grams of carbohydrates.
Beans-black, 6 oz., 227 calories, 15 grams of protein, 1 gram of fat, 41 grams of carbohydrates.
Beans-black-eyed peas, 1 cup, 184 calories, 15 grams of protein, 1 gram of fat, 41 grams of carbohydrates.

Beans-chickpeas, 1 cup, 285 calories, 12 grams of protein, 3 grams of fat, 54 grams of carbohydrates.

Beans-fava beans, 1/2 cup, 94 calories, 6 grams of protein, 0 fat, 17 grams of carbohydrates.

Beans-great northern, 1 cup, 299 calories, 19 grams of protein, 1 gram of fat, 55 grams of carbohydrates.

Beans-kidney, 1/2 cup, 108 calories, 7 grams of protein, 1 gram of fat, 19 grams of carbohydrates.

Beans-lima, 1/2 cup, 95 calories, 6 grams of protein, 6 grams of fat, 18 grams of carbohydrates.

Beans-navy, 1 cup, 296 calories, 20 grams of protein, 1 gram of fat, 54 grams of carbohydrates.

Beans-white, 1 cup, 300 calories, 20 grams of protein, 1 gram of fat, 55 grams of carbohydrates.

Beef-brisket, braised, 3 oz., 200 calories, 32 grams of protein, 9 grams of fat, 0 carbohydrates.

Beef-chuck, braised, 3 oz., 300 calories, 27 grams of protein, 24 grams of fat, 0 carbohydrates.

Beef-eye round, roasted, 4 oz., 190 calories, 33 grams of protein, 5 grams of fat, 0 carbohydrates.

Beef-ground, 80% lean, broiled, 3 oz., 234 calories, 22 grams of protein, 15 grams of fat, 0 carbohydrates.

Beef-jerky, 1 oz., 122 calories, 10 grams of protein, 8 grams of fat, 3 grams of carbohydrates.

Beef-London broil, broiled, 4 oz., 260 calories, 35 grams of protein, 12 grams of fat, 0 carbohydrates.

Beef-NY strip, broiled, 4 oz., 219 calories, 33 grams of protein, 9 grams of fat, 0 carbohydrates.

Beef-porterhouse steak, broiled, 8 oz., 625 calories, 55 grams of protein, 44 grams of fat, 0 carbohydrates.

Beef-rib eye, broiled, 4 oz., 221 calories, 34 grams of protein, 9 grams of fat, 0 carbohydrates.

Beef-skirt steak, broiled, 4 oz., 289 calories, 27 grams of protein, 19 grams of fat, 0 carbohydrates.

Beef-T-bone steak, broiled, 8 oz., 600 calories, 35 grams of protein, 40 grams of fat, 0 carbohydrates.

Beer-regular, 12 oz., 153 calories, 2 grams of protein, 0 fat, 13 grams of carbohydrates.

Biscuits-buttermilk, 3 biscuits, 150 calories, 4 grams of protein, 2 grams of fat, 29 grams of carbohydrates.

Blackberries-fresh, 1/2 cup, 31 calories, 1 gram of protein, 0 fat, 7 grams of carbohydrates.

Blueberries-fresh, 1/2 cup, 41 calories, 1 gram of protein, 0 fat, 11 grams of carbohydrates.

Bread-regular, 1 slice, 88 calories, 3 grams of protein, 1 gram of protein, 17 grams of carbohydrates.

Bread-rye, 1 slice, 83 calories, 3 grams of protein, 1 gram of fat, 15 grams of carbohydrates.

Bread-seven grain, 1 slice, 80 calories, 3 grams of protein, 1 gram of fat, 15 grams of carbohydrates.

Bread-whole wheat, 1 slice, 69 calories, 3 grams of protein, 1 gram of fat, 13 grams of carbohydrates.

Bread-low calorie, 60 calories, 3 grams of protein, 1 gram of fat, 12 grams of carbohydrates.

Bread-stick, 1 stick, 41 calories, 1 gram of protein, 1 gram of fat, 7 grams of carbohydrates.

Broccoli-cooked, 3 oz., 30 calories, 2 grams of protein, 0 fat, 6 grams of carbohydrates.

Broccoli rabe-cooked, 3 oz., 28 calories, 3 grams of protein, 0 fat, 3 grams of carbohydrates.

Brussel sprouts-cooked, 6 sprouts, 45 calories, 3 grams of protein, 1 gram of fat, 9 grams of carbohydrates.

Buckwheat-cooked, 6 oz., 155 calories, 7 grams of protein, 1 gram of fat, 33 grams of carbohydrates.

Buffalo-roast, 4 oz., 150 calories, 22 grams of protein, 7 grams of fat, 0 carbohydrates.

Bison-roasted, 4 oz., 150 calories, 22 grams of protein, 7 grams of fat, 0 carbohydrates.

Bulgur-cooked, 1/2 cup, 76 calories, 3 grams of protein, 0 fat, 17 grams of carbohydrates.

Butter, 1 tbsp., 102 calories, 0 protein, 12 grams of fat, 0 carbohydrates.

Cabbage, 1 cup, 35 calories, 3 grams of protein, 0 fat, 8 grams of carbohydrates.

Cake-chocolate mousse, 2 oz., 150 calories, 3 grams of protein, 7 grams of fat, 17 grams of carbohydrates.

Cake-apple turnover, 6 oz., 600 calories, 7 grams of protein, 34 grams of fat, 83 grams of carbohydrates.

Cake-banana, 3 oz., 350 calories, 5 grams of protein, 23 grams of fat, 29 grams of carbohydrates.

Cake-Boston cream, 3 oz., 230 calories, 2 grams of protein, 8 grams of fat, 39 grams of carbohydrates.

Cake-brownie, 2 oz., 227 calories, 3 grams of protein, 9 grams of fat, 36 grams of carbohydrates.

Cake-cheesecake, 4 oz., 400 calories, 10 grams of protein, 25 grams of fat, 37 grams of carbohydrates.

Cake-fruit cake, 2 oz., 150 calories, 1 gram of protein, 4 grams of fat, 26 grams of carbohydrates.

Cake-funnel cake, 3 oz., 270 calories, 7 grams of protein, 14 grams of fat, 29 grams of carbohydrates.

Cake-jelly roll, 2 oz., 146 calories, 3 grams of protein, 2 grams of fat, 28 grams of carbohydrates.

Cake-pound cake, 1 oz., 120 calories, 2 grams of protein, 5 grams of fat, 15 grams of carbohydrates.

Cake-apple strudel, 2 oz., 170 calories, 2 grams of protein, 7 grams of fat, 26 grams of carbohydrates.

Candy-jelly beans, 1 oz., 104 calories, 0 protein, 0 fat, 26 grams of carbohydrates.

Candy-milk chocolate, 2 oz., 300 calories, 4 grams of protein, 16 grams of fat, 30 grams of carbohydrates.

Cantaloupe, 1 cup, 57 calories, 1 gram of protein, 0 fat, 13 grams of carbohydrates.

Capers, 1 tbsp., 2 calories, 0 protein, 0 fat, 0 carbohydrates.

Carrots-cooked, 1/2 cup, 35 calories, 1 gram of protein, 8 grams of carbohydrates.

Cauliflower-cooked, 2 oz., 12 calories, 1 gram of protein, 0 fat, 2 grams of carbohydrates.

Celery, 2 oz., 10 calories, 0 protein, 0 fat, 2 grams of carbohydrates.

Cereal-corn flakes, 1 cup, 100 calories, 2 grams of protein, 0 fat, 23 grams of carbohydrates.

Cereal-oatmeal, cooked, 6 oz., 150 calories, 5 grams of protein, 2 grams of fat, 19 grams of carbohydrates.

Cereal-granola, 2 oz., 200 calories, 6 grams of protein, 3 grams of fat, 39 grams of carbohydrates.

Cereal-farina, 1 cup, 120 calories, 3 grams of protein, 0 fat, 22 grams of carbohydrates.

Cheese-American, 1 oz., 93 calories, 6 grams of protein, 18 grams of carbohydrates.

Cheese-brie, 1 oz., 95 calories, 8 grams of protein, 8 grams of fat, 0 carbohydrates.

Cheese-cheddar, 1 oz., 114 calories, 7 grams of protein, 9 grams of fat, 0 carbohydrates.

Cheese-Colby, 1 oz., 112 calories, 7 grams of protein, 9 grams of fat, 1 gram of carbohydrates.

Cheese-cottage, 1/2 cup, 100 calories, 13 grams of protein, 5 grams of fat, 4 grams of carbohydrates.

Cheese-cream cheese, 1 oz., 99 calories, 2 grams of protein, 10 grams of fat, 1 gram of carbohydrates.

Cheese-edam, 1 oz., 115 calories, 12 grams of protein, 5 grams of fat, 0 carbohydrates.

Cheese-feta, 1 oz., 75 calories, 4 grams of protein, 6 grams of fat, 1 gram of carbohydrates.

Cheese-gorgonzola, 1 oz., 107 calories, 5 grams of protein, 9 grams of fat, 0 carbohydrates.

Cheese-gruyere, 1 oz., 117 calories, 8 grams of protein, 9 grams of fat, 0 carbohydrates.

Cheese-low fat, 1 oz., 49 calories, 7 grams of protein, 2 grams of fat, 1 gram of carbohydrates.

Cheese-monetary, 1 oz., 106 calories, 7 grams of protein, 9 grams of fat, 0 carbohydrates.

Cheese-mozzarella, 1 oz., 80 calories, 6 grams of protein, 6 grams of fat, 1 gram of carbohydrates.

Cheese-mozzarella, fresh, 1 oz., 80 calories, 6 grams of protein, 6 grams of fat, 0 carbohydrates.

Cheese-mozzarella, part skim, 1 oz., 72 calories, 7 grams of protein, 7 grams of fat, 1 gram of carbohydrates.

Cheese-parmesan, 1 oz., 111 calories, 10 grams of protein, 7 grams of fat, 1 gram of carbohydrates.

Cheese-provolone, 1 oz., 100 calories, 7 grams of protein, 8 grams of fat, 1 gram of carbohydrates.
Cheese-ricotta, whole milk, 4 oz., 202 calories, 12 grams of protein, 14 grams of fat, 4 grams of carbohydrates.
Cheese-swiss, 1 oz., 110 calories, 8 grams of protein, 8 grams of fat, 0 carbohydrates.
Cherries-fresh, 20 cherries, 86 calories, 1 gram of protein, 1 gram of fat, 22 grams of carbohydrates.
Chestnuts-roasted, 1 oz., 57 calories, 1 gram of protein, 0 grams of fat, 13 grams of carbohydrates.
Chia seeds, 1 oz., 134 calories, 5 grams of protein, 7 grams of fat, 14 grams of carbohydrates.
Chicken-breast, roasted, 3 oz., 147 calories, 27 grams of protein, 3 grams of fat, 0 carbohydrates.
Chicory, 1/2 cup, 4 calories, 0 protein, 0 fat, 1 gram of carbohydrates.
Chili with beans, 9 oz., 270 calories, 18 grams of protein, 8 grams of fat, 35 grams of carbohydrates.
Chili-vegetarian, 9 oz., 200 calories, 13 grams of protein, 1 gram of fat, 37 grams of carbohydrates.
Chips-banana, fried, 1 oz., 147 calories, 1 gram of protein, 10 grams of fat, 17 grams of carbohydrates.
Chips-corn, fried, 1 oz., 147 calories, 2 grams of protein, 8 grams of fat, 18 grams of carbohydrates.
Chips-potato, fried, 1 oz., 155 calories, 2 grams of protein, 11 grams of fat, 14 grams of carbohydrates.
Chutney-mango, 3 oz., 227 calories, 2 grams of protein, 5 grams of fat, 43 grams of carbohydrates.
Cilantro-fresh, 1/4cup, 1 calorie, 0 protein, 0 fat, 0 carbohydrates.
Cocoa, 1 tbsp., 10 calories, 0 protein, 1 gram of fat, 3 grams of carbohydrates.
Coconut-fresh, 1 oz., 100 calories, 1 gram of protein, 10 grams of fat, 4 grams of carbohydrates.
Coconut-water, 1/2 cup, 23 calories, 1 gram of protein, 0 fat, 4 grams of carbohydrates.
Coconut-cream, sweetened, 1/2 cup, 264 calories, 1 gram of protein, 12 grams of fat, 39 grams of carbohydrates.

Coffee-plain, 8 oz., 2 calories, 0 protein, 0 fat, 0 carbohydrates.

Coffee-cappuccino, 8 oz., 77 calories, 4 grams of protein, 4 grams of fat, 6 grams of carbohydrates.

Coffee-espresso, 4 oz., 2 calories, 0 protein, 0 fat, 0 carbohydrates.

Collard greens, boiled, 1/2 cup, 17 calories, 1 gram of protein, 0 fat, 4 grams of carbohydrates.

Cookie-chocolate chip, 1 cookie, 79 calories, 1 gram of protein, 4 grams of fat, 10 grams of carbohydrates.

Cookie-oatmeal, 1 cookie, 74 calories, 1 gram of protein, 3 grams of fat, 10 grams of carbohydrates.

Cookie-animal cracker, 1 cookie, 11calories, 0 protein, 0 fat, 2 grams of carbohydrates.

Cookie-ginger snap, 1 cookie, 29 calories, 0 protein, 1 gram of fat, 5 grams of carbohydrates.

Cookie-graham cracker, 1 cracker, 30 calories, 1 gram of protein, 1 gram of fat, 5 grams of carbohydrates.

Cookie-biscotti, 1 biscotti, 110 calories, 2 grams of protein, 5 grams of fat, 17 grams of carbohydrates.

Corn-canned, sweet, 3 oz., 70 calories, 2 grams of protein, 2 grams of fat, 15 grams of carbohydrates.

Corn on the cob, 1 cob, boiled, 90 calories, 2 grams of protein, 0 fat, 14 grams of carbohydrates.

Corn-meal, cooked,1 cup, 223 calories, 5 grams of protein, 1 gram of fat, 47 grams of carbohydrates.

Cream-half and half, 1 cup, 317 calories, 7 grams of protein, 28 grams of fat, 10 grams of carbohydrates.

Cream-heavy, 1tbsp., 52 calories, 0 protein, 6 grams of fat, 0 carbohydrates.

Cream-sour, 1/2 cup,125 calories, 2 grams of protein, 24 grams of fat, 4 grams of carbohydrates.

Crepes-plain, 1 crepe, 112 calories, 4 grams of protein, 6 grams of fat, 11 grams of carbohydrates.

Croissant-butter, 2 oz., 250 calories, 4 grams of protein, 12 grams of fat, 30 grams of carbohydrates.

Cucumber-fresh, 7 oz., 24 calories, 1 gram of protein, 0 fat, 4 grams of carbohydrates.

Currants-fresh, 1/2 cup, 36 calories, 1 gram of protein, 0 fat, 9 grams of carbohydrates.

Custard, 4 oz., 130 calories, 7 grams of protein, 3 grams of fat, 19 grams of carbohydrates.

Dates, 1 oz., 100 calories, 1 gram of protein, 0 fat, 30 grams of carbohydrates.

Deli meat-bologna,1 oz., 87 calories, 4 grams of protein, 7 grams of fat, 2 grams of carbohydrates.

Deli meat-mortadella,1/2 oz., 47 calories, 2 grams of protein, 4 grams of fat, 0 carbohydrates.

Deli meat-olive loaf, 2 oz., 134 calories, 7 grams of protein, 9 grams of fat, 5 grams of carbohydrates.

Deli meat-pastrami, 1 oz., 41 calories, 6 grams of protein, 2 grams of fat, 0 carbohydrates.

Deli meat-peperoni, 1 oz., 135 calories, 6 grams of protein, 12 grams of fat, 1 gram of carbohydrates.

Deli meat-salami, 1 oz., 113 calories, 4 grams of protein, 9 grams of fat, 2 grams of carbohydrates.

Doughnut-old fashioned, 1 doughnut, 226 calories, 3 grams of protein, 13 grams of fat, 25 grams of carbohydrates.

Doughnut-cream filled, 1 doughnut, 307 calories, 5 grams of protein, 21 grams of fat, 26 grams of carbohydrates.

Doughnut-jelly filled, 1 doughnut, 289 calories, 5 grams of protein, 16 grams of fat, 33 grams of carbohydrates.

Duck-boneless, 8 oz., 450 calories, 52 grams of protein, 30 grams of fat, 0 carbohydrates.

Egg-hardboiled, 1 egg, 80 calories, 6 grams of protein, 5 grams of fat, 1 gram of carbohydrates.

Eggs-benedict, 2 eggs, 625 calories, 35 grams of protein, 45 grams of fat, 26 grams of carbohydrates.

Egg-poached, 1 egg, 71 calories, 6 grams of protein, 5 grams of fat, 1 gram of carbohydrates.

Eggs-western omelet, 3 eggs, 355 calories, 24 grams of protein, 23 grams of fat, 6 grams of carbohydrates.

Egg-whites, 3 egg whites, poached, 50 calories, 12 grams of protein, 0 fat, 1 gram of carbohydrates.

Egg roll-pork and shrimp, 1 roll, 185 calories, 8 grams of protein, 4 grams of fat, 20 grams of carbohydrates.

English muffin, 1 muffin, 129 calories, 5 grams of protein, 1 gram of fat, 25 grams of carbohydrates.

Fat-lard, 1 tbsp., 115 calories, 0 protein, 13 grams of fat, 0 carbohydrates.

Fat-shortening, 1 tbsp., 110 calories, 0 grams of protein, 12 grams of fat, 0 carbohydrates.

Fennel-fresh, 1 cup, 27 calories, 1 gram of protein, 0 fat, 6 grams of carbohydrates.

Figs, 1 fig, 21 calories, 0 protein, 0 fat, 5 grams of carbohydrates.

Fish-bass, 4 oz., 205 calories, 32 grams of protein, 9 grams of fat, 0 carbohydrates.

Fish-calamari, fried, 3 oz., 320 calories, 11 grams of protein, 12 grams of fat, 25 grams of carbohydrates.

Fish-caviar, 2 tsp., 81 calories, 8 grams of protein, 6 grams of fat, 1 gram of carbohydrates.

Fish-clams, fresh, baked, 10 medium, 155 calories, 25 grams of protein, 2 grams of fat, 5 grams of carbohydrates.

Fish-cod, broiled, 3 oz., 89 calories, 19 grams of protein, 1 gram of fat, 0 carbohydrates.

Fish-crab, 1 Dungeness crab, steamed,140 calories, 28 grams of protein, 2 grams of fat, 1 gram of carbohydrates.

Fish-cray fish, 3 oz., boiled, 97 calories, 20 grams of protein, 1 gram of fat, 0 carbohydrates.

Fish-flounder, broiled, 4 oz., 140 calories, 28 grams of protein, 2 grams of fat, 0 carbohydrates.

Fish-grouper, 3 oz., broiled, 100 calories, 21 grams of protein, 1 gram of fat, 0 carbohydrates.

Fish-haddock, broiled, 4 oz., 127 calories, 27 grams of protein, 1 gram of fat, 0 carbohydrates.

Fish-halibut, broiled, 3 oz., 203 calories, 16 grams of protein, 15 grams of fat, 0 carbohydrates.

Fish-lobster, broiled, 3 oz., 83 calories, 17 grams of protein, 1 gram of fat, 2 grams of carbohydrates.

Fish-mahi-mahi, broiled, 4 oz., 192 calories, 18 grams of protein, 13 grams of fat, 1 gram of carbohydrates.

Fish-millet, grilled, 6 oz., 207 calories, 6 grams of protein, 2 grams of fat, 4 grams of carbohydrates.

Fish-mussels, steamed, 3 oz., 147 calories, 20 grams of protein, 4 grams of fat, 6 grams of carbohydrates.

Fish-oysters, raw, 6 oysters, 175 calories, 8 grams of protein, 11 gram of fat, 10 grams of carbohydrates.

Fish-salmon, broiled, 4 oz., 235 calories, 24 grams of protein, 15 grams of fat, 0 carbohydrates.

Fish-salmon, smoked, 1 oz., 35 calories, 5 grams of protein, 2 grams of fat, 0 carbohydrates.

Fish-shark steak, broiled, 3 oz., 195 calories, 16 grams of protein, 12 grams of fat, 5 grams of carbohydrates.

Fish-shrimp, jumbo broiled, 1 oz., 45 calories, 8 grams of protein, 1 gram of fat, 0 carbohydrates.

Fish-shrimp, large steamed, 1 oz., 55 calories, 6 grams of protein, 1 gram of fat, 0 carbohydrates.

Fish-snapper, broiled, 6 oz., 222 calories, 47 grams of protein, 2 grams of fat, 0 carbohydrates.

Fish-swordfish, broiled, 3 oz., 135 calories, 25 grams of protein, 5 grams of fat, 0 carbohydrates.

Fish-tuna steak, grilled, 3 oz., 120 calories, 27 grams of protein, 1 gram of fat, 0 carbohydrates.

Fish-tuna, canned in water, 1 oz., 35 calories, 6 grams of protein, 1 gram of fat, 1 gram of carbohydrates.

Flax seeds, 1 oz., 140 calories, 6 grams of protein, 9 grams of fat, 9 grams of carbohydrates.

Flour-wheat, all purpose, 1/2 cup, 228 calories, 6 grams of protein, 1 gram of fat, 48 grams of carbohydrates.

Flour-chickpea, 1/2 cup, 178 calories, 10 grams of protein, 3 grams of fat, 27 grams of carbohydrates.

Flour-soy, 1/2 cup, 92 calories, 7 grams of protein, 4 grams of fat, 7 grams of carbohydrates.

Flour-almond, 2 tbsp., 80 calories, 4 grams of protein, 5 grams of fat, 5 grams of carbohydrates.

Fruit juice-apple, 1 cup, 113 calories, 0 protein, 0 fat, 0 carbohydrates.

Fruit juice-orange, 1 cup, 111 calories, 2 grams of protein, 0 fat, 26 grams of carbohydrates.

Fruit juice-grapefruit, 1 cup, 96 calories, 1 gram of protein, 0 fat, 23 grams of carbohydrates.

Fruit juice-grape, 8 oz., 150 calories, 0 protein, 0 fat, 40 grams of carbohydrates.

Fruit juice-pomegranate, 8 oz., 130 calories, 0 protein, 0 fat, 30 grams of carbohydrates.

Goat-roasted, 3 oz., 122 calories, 23 grams of protein, 3 grams of fat, 0 carbohydrates.

Grape leaves, stuffed with rice, 2 oz., 92 calories, 1 gram of protein, 3 grams of fat, 8 grams of carbohydrates.

Grapefruit, 1/2 grapefruit, 52 calories, 1 gram of protein, 0 fat, 13 grams of carbohydrates.

Guava-fresh, 1 fruit, 45 calories, 1 gram of protein, 1 gram of fat, 11 grams of carbohydrates.

Ham-boneless, roasted, 3 oz., 130 calories, 18 grams of protein, 5 grams of fat, 1 gram of carbohydrates.

Hamburger with cheese and bun, 5 oz., 350 calories, 17 grams of protein, 17 grams of fat, 28 grams of carbohydrates.

Hominy-canned, 1 cup, 119 calories, 2 grams of protein, 1 gram of fat, 24 grams of carbohydrates.

Honey, 1 tbsp., 64 calories, 0 protein, 0 fat, 17 grams of carbohydrates.

Honeydew-fresh, 1 cup, 61 calories, 1 gram of protein, 0 fat, 15 grams of carbohydrates.

Horseradish, 1 tsp., 0 protein, 0 fat, 0 carbohydrates.

Hot chocolate, 8 oz., 209 calories, 9 grams of protein, 1 gram of fat, 30 grams of carbohydrates.

Hotdog on bun, 242 calories, 10 grams of protein, 15 grams of fat, 18 grams of carbohydrates.

Hotdog on bun with chili, 297 calories, 14 grams of protein, 13 grams of fat, 31 grams of carbohydrates.

Hotdog-corn dog, 460 calories, 17 grams of protein, 19 grams of fat, 56 grams of carbohydrates.

Hotdog-tofu dog, 45 calories, 8 grams of protein, 1 gram of fat, 2 grams of carbohydrates.

Hot sauce, 1 tsp, 3 calories, 0 protein, 0 fat, 0 carbohydrates.

Ice-cream-chocolate, 4 oz., 143 calories. 3 grams of protein, 7 grams of fat, 19 grams of carbohydrates.

Ice-creme-vanilla, 4 oz., 132 calories, 2 grams of protein, 7 grams of fat, 16 grams of carbohydrates.
Ice-cream sandwich, 220 calories, 4 grams of protein, 10 grams of fat, 30 grams of carbohydrates.
Ice pop, 100% fruit juice, 8 oz., 54 calories, 0 protein, 0 fat, 13 grams of carbohydrates.
Jelly, 1tbsp., 51 calories, 0 protein, 0 fat, 13 grams of carbohydrates.
Ketchup, 1 tbsp., 19 calories, 0 protein, 0 fat, 2 grams of carbohydrates.
Knish-potato, 5 oz., 180 calories, 7 grams of protein, 6 grams of fat, 30 grams of carbohydrates.
Lambchops, 4 oz., roasted, 222 calories, 17 grams of protein, 16 grams of fat, 0 carbohydrates.
Lemon, 4 oz., 22 calories, 1 gram of protein, 0 fat, 12 grams of carbohydrates.
Lentils-cooked, 1 cup, 230 calories, 18 grams of protein, 1 gram of fat, 40 grams of carbohydrates.
Lettuce-arugula, 1 oz., 8 calories, 0 protein, 0 fat, 0 carbohydrates.
Lettuce-iceberg, 1 oz., 5 calories, 0 protein, 0 fat, 1gram of carbohydrates.
Lettuce-red leaf, 4 oz., 18 calories, 1 gram of protein, 0 fat, 32 grams of carbohydrates.
Lettuce-romaine, 1 oz., 4 calories, 0 protein, 0 fat, 1 gram of carbohydrates.
Lime-one fruit, 20 calories, 0 protein, 0 fat, 7 grams of carbohydrates.
Mango-fresh, 7 oz., 130 calories, 1 gram of protein, 1 gram of fat, 35 grams of carbohydrates.
Margarine, 1 tbsp., 1000 calories, 0 protein, 11 grams of fat, 0 carbohydrates.
Marshmallow, one each, 23 calories, 0 protein, 0 fat, 6 grams of carbohydrates.
Mayonnaise, 1tbsp., 99 calories, 0 protein, 11 grams of fat, 1 gram of carbohydrates.
Meatball, 1 oz., 74 calories, 7 grams of protein, 5 grams of fat, 3 grams of carbohydrates.
Milk-whole milk, 1 cup, 148 calories, 8 grams of protein, 8 grams of

fat, 12 grams of carbohydrates.

Milk-chocolate, 1 cup, 208 calories, 8 grams of protein, 8 grams of fat, 26 grams of carbohydrates.

Milk-almond, 1 cup, 39 calories, 2 grams of protein, 3 grams of fat, 2 grams of carbohydrates.

Millet, 6 oz., 207 calories, 6 grams of protein, 2 grams of fat, 41 grams of carbohydrates.

Mushrooms-maitake, 1 cup, 26 calories, 1 gram of protein, 0 fat, 5 grams of carbohydrates.

Mushrooms-morel, 4 oz., 12 calories, 2 grams of protein, 0 fat, 8 grams of carbohydrates.

Mushrooms-oyster, 1 cup, 30 calories, 3 grams of protein, 0 fat, 2 grams of carbohydrates.

Mushrooms-portobello, 3 oz., 22 calories, 2 grams of protein, 0 fat, 4 grams of carbohydrates.

Mushrooms-shitake, 3 oz., 50 calories, 1 gram of protein, 0 fat, 10 grams of carbohydrates.

Mustard-brown, 1 tsp., 5 calories, 0 protein, 0 fat, 0 carbohydrates.

Mustard-greens, 1 cup, boiled, 21 calories, 3 grams of protein, 0 fat, 3 grams of carbohydrates.

Nectarine, 1 fruit, 69 calories, 2 grams of protein, 1 gram of fat, 16 grams of carbohydrates.

Noodles-egg, 1 cup, 145 calories, 5 grams of protein, 2 grams of fat, 27 grams of carbohydrates.

Noodles-soba, 4 oz., 113 calories, 6 grams of protein, 0 fat, 24 grams of carbohydrates.

Noodles-tofu, 2 oz., 20 calories, 1 gram of protein, 1 gram of fat, 3 grams of carbohydrates.

Nuts-almonds, 1 oz., 163 calories, 6 grams of protein, 14 grams of fat, 6 grams of carbohydrates.

Nuts-brazil, 1 oz., 186 calories, 4 grams of protein, 17 grams of fat, 0 carbohydrates.

Nuts-cashews, 18 nuts, 160 calories, 4 grams of protein, 13 grams of fat, 9 grams of carbohydrates.

Nuts-hazelnuts, 1/4 cup, 210 calories, 5 grams of protein, 20 grams of fat, 6 grams of carbohydrates.

Nuts-macadamia, 11 nuts, 200 calories, 2 grams of protein, 22 grams of fat, 4 grams of carbohydrates.

Nuts-pistachio, 1 oz., dry roasted, 161 calories, 6 grams of protein, 13 grams of fat, 8 grams of carbohydrates.

Nuts-peanuts, dry roasted, 1/4 cup, 203 calories, 6 grams of protein, 18 grams of fat, 9 grams of carbohydrates.

Nuts-pecan, dry roasted, 1 oz., 187 calories, 2 grams of protein, 18 grams of fat, 6 grams of carbohydrates.

Nuts-pine nuts, 1/4 cup, 277 calories, 5 grams of protein, 23 grams of fat, 4 grams of carbohydrates.

Nuts-walnuts, 1/4 cup, 180 calories, 5 grams of protein, 5 grams of fat, 4 grams of carbohydrates.

Oils from vegetables and fruits, Olive, palm, corn, canola, etc., are similar in the basic nutritional value. 1 tbsp., 120 calories, 0 protein, 14 grams of fat, 0 carbohydrates.

Olives-black, one olive, 4 calories, 0 protein, 0 fat, 0 carbohydrates.

Olives-Greek, 1 olive, 16 calories, 0 protein, 1 gram of fat, 1 gram of carbohydrates.

Olives-green, 1 olive, 5 calories, 0 protein, 0 fat, 0 carbohydrates.

Onion, 1 tbsp., 4 calories, 0 protein, 0 fat, 5 grams of carbohydrates.

Pancake-buttermilk, 4 oz., 240 calories, 6 grams of protein, 4 grams of fat, 47 grams of carbohydrates.

Pancake-syrup, 1/4 cup, 209 calories, 0 protein, 0 fat, 55 grams of carbohydrates.

Papaya, 1 cup, 55 calories, 1 gram of protein, 0 fat, 14 grams of carbohydrates.

Passion fruit, 1/2 cup, 114 calories, 3 grams of protein, 1 gram of fat, 28 grams of carbohydrates.

Pasta-cooked, plain, 1 cup, 197 calories, 7 grams of protein, 1 gram of fat, 40 grams of carbohydrates.

Peach-fresh, 1 fruit, 58 calories. 1 gram of protein, 0 fat, 14 grams of carbohydrates.

Peanut butter, 2 tbsp., 188 calories, 8 grams of protein, 16 grams of fat, 7 grams of carbohydrates.

Pear-fresh, 1 fruit, 133 calories, 1 gram of protein, 0 fat, 36 grams of carbohydrates.

Peas-canned, 1/2 cup, 66 calories, 4 grams of protein, 0 fat, 12 grams of carbohydrates.

Peppers-sweet, 3 oz., 23 calories, 1 gram of protein, 0 fat, 5 grams of carbohydrates.

Pepper-hot, habanero, 1 tbsp., 9 calories, 1 gram of protein, 0 fat, 2 grams of carbohydrates.

Persimmons-fresh, 6 oz., 118 calories, 1 gram of protein, 0 fat, 31 grams of carbohydrates.

Pickle-dill, 5 oz., 26 calories, 1 gram of protein, 0 fat, 7 grams of carbohydrates.

Pierogi, potato and onion, 4 oz., 160 calories, 5 grams of protein, 2 grams of fat, 32 grams of carbohydrates.

Pineapple-fresh, 3 oz., 42 calories, 0 protein, 0 fat, 11 grams of carbohydrates.

Pizza-tomato and cheese, 6 oz., 300 calories, 15 grams of protein, 10 grams of fat, 45 grams of carbohydrates.

Popcorn, air popped, 1 cup, 31 calories, 1 gram of protein, 0 fat, 6 grams of carbohydrates.

Pork-loin, broiled, 4 oz., 220 calories, 30 grams of protein, 11 grams of fat, 0 carbohydrates.

Pork-ribs, grilled, 4 oz., 300 calories, 16 grams of protein, 24 grams of fat, 4 grams of carbohydrates.

Potato-baked, 6 oz., 200 calories, 5 grams of protein, 0 fat, 53 grams of carbohydrates.

Potatoes-fries, 3 oz, 120 calories, 1 gram of protein, 5 grams of fat, 16 grams of carbohydrates.

Potatoes-mashed, 1/2 cup, 150 calories, 3 grams of protein, 7 grams of fat, 20 grams of carbohydrates.

Potatoes-sweet potato, baked, 165 calories, 4 grams of protein, 0 fat, 35 grams of carbohydrates.

Pretzels-hard, 2 oz., 229 calories, 5 grams of protein, 2 grams of fat, 48 grams of carbohydrates.

Pretzels-soft, 5 oz., 483 carbohydrates, 12 grams of protein, 4 grams of fat, 90 grams of carbohydrates.

Pudding-chocolate, 4 oz., 140 calories, 4 grams of protein, 4 grams of fat, 24 grams of carbohydrates.

Pudding-tapioca, 4 oz., 130 calories, 3 grams of protein, 3 grams of fat, 23 grams of carbohydrates.

Pudding-rice, 4 oz., 135 calories, 4 grams of protein, 4 grams of fat,

21 grams of carbohydrates.

Pudding-soy, 5 oz., 130 calories, 5 grams of protein, 3 grams of fat, 25 grams of carbohydrates.

Pumpkin seeds, 1/4 cup, 190 calories, 10 grams of protein, 15 grams of fat, 5 grams of carbohydrates.

Quinoa, cooked, 1 cup, 225 calories, 7 grams of protein, 6 grams of fat, 40 grams of carbohydrates.

Radicchio, 1/2 cup, 5 calories, 0 protein, 0 fat, 2 grams of carbohydrates.

Raisins-seedless, 1/4 cup, 110 calories, 1 gram of protein, 0 fat, 31 grams of carbohydrates.

Raspberries-fresh, 1 pt., 172 calories, 5 grams of protein, 1 gram of fat, 35 grams of carbohydrates.

Rice-arborio, boiled, 1/2 cup, 100 calories, 2 grams of protein, 0 fat, 21 grams of carbohydrates.

Rice-brown, boiled, 6 oz., 200 calories, 5 grams of protein, 3 grams of fat, 43 grams of carbohydrates.

Rice-white, long grain, boiled, 5 oz., 200 calories, 5 grams of protein, 0 fat, 42 grams of carbohydrates.

Rice-basmati, boiled, 1 cup, 206 calories, 8 grams of protein, 2 grams of fat, 90 grams of carbohydrates.

Rice-wild, boiled, 4 oz., 120 calories, 5 grams of protein, 0 fat, 25 grams of carbohydrates.

Sauerkraut, 1 oz., 6 calories, 0 protein, 0 fat, 1 gram of carbohydrates.

Sausage-pork, 2 oz., broiled, 195 calories, 7 grams of protein, 15grams of fat, 1 gram of carbohydrates.

Sausage-bratwurst, 3 oz., cooked, 235 calories, 11 grams of protein, 20 grams of fat, 3 grams of carbohydrates.

Sausage- chorizo, 2 oz., 270 calories, 12 grams of protein, 25 grams of fat, 1 gram of carbohydrates.

Sausage-Italian, cooked, 2 oz., 227 calories, 12 grams of protein, 18 grams of fat, 2 grams of carbohydrates.

Sausage-knockwurst, cooked, 3 oz., 235 calories, 9 grams of protein, 22 grams of fat, 2 grams of carbohydrates.

Sausage-kielbasa, cooked, 2 oz., 132 calories, 6 grams of protein, 12 grams of fat, 2 grams of carbohydrates.

Seaweed, 1 oz., 11 calories, 0 protein, 0 fat, 2 grams of carbohydrates.

Sesame-seeds, 1 tsp., 15 calories, 1 gram of protein, 2 grams of fat, 1 gram of carbohydrates.

Sesame-tahini, 1 tbsp., 88 calories, 3 grams of protein, 6 grams of fat, 3 grams of carbohydrates.

Sherbet-orange, 1/2 cup, 137 calories, 1 gram of protein, 1 gram of fat, 28 grams of carbohydrates.

Soy-beans, cooked, 1/2 cup, 130 calories, 10 grams of protein, 5 grams of fat, 9 grams of carbohydrates.

Soy-beans, sprouts, 1/2 cup, 40 calories, 5 grams of protein, 2 grams of fat, 2 grams of carbohydrates.

Soy-sauce, 1 tbsp., 7 calories, 0 protein, 0 fat, 1 gram of carbohydrates.

Spinach-raw, 1 oz., 5 calories, 0 protein, 1 gram of fat, 1 gram of carbohydrates.

Strawberries-fresh, 1 cup, 55 calories, 1 gram of protein, 0 fat, 10 grams of carbohydrates.

Sugar-white, 1 tbsp., 48 calories, 0 protein, 0 fat, 2 grams of carbohydrates.

Sugar-dark brown, 1 tsp., 15 calories, 0 protein, 0 fat, 4 grams of carbohydrates.

Swiss chard, cooked, 1/2 cup, 19 calories, 2 grams of protein, 0 fat, 5 grams of carbohydrates.

Tofu-soy-firm, 3 oz., 120 calories, 15 grams of protein, 6 grams of fat, 3 grams of carbohydrates.

Tomato-crushed, canned, 1/4 cup, 20 calories, 1 gram of protein, 0 fat, 5 grams of carbohydrates.

Tomato-fresh, 1 tomato, 25 calories, 1 gram of protein, 0 fat, 4 grams of carbohydrates.

Tomato-puree, canned, 9 oz., 100 calories, 5 grams of protein, 1 gram of fat, 25 grams of carbohydrates.

Tomato-sauce, canned, 9 oz., 60 calories, 3 grams of protein, 14 grams of carbohydrates.

Tomato-whole, peeled, canned, 1/2 cup, 22 calories, 1 gram of protein, 0 fat, 5 grams of carbohydrates.

Turkey-breast, 1 oz., 35 calories, 6 grams of protein, 0 fat, 0 carbohydrates.

<u>Water chestnuts</u>, 1/2 cup, 26 calories, 1 gram of protein, 0 fat, 6 grams of carbohydrates.

<u>Wine-red</u>, 5 oz., 130 calories, 0 protein, 0 fat, 5 grams of carbohydrates.

<u>Wine-white</u>, 5 oz., 120 calories, 0 protein, 0 fat, 4 grams of carbohydrates.

<u>Vinegar-white</u>, 1 tsp., 5 calories, 0 protein, 0 fat, 0 carbohydrates.

<u>Wrap-tortilla</u>, low fat, 50 calories, 4 grams of protein, 2 grams of fat, 16 grams of carbohydrates.

<u>Yogurt-plain</u>, whole milk, 8 oz., 140 calories, 7 grams of protein, 7 grams of fat, 12 grams of carbohydrates.

<u>Zucchini,</u> roasted, 4 oz., 20 calories, 1 gram of protein, 0 fat, 5 grams of carbohydrates.

Recipes

Here are a few recipes for sandwiches, tortilla wraps, and lettuce wraps. These recipes can easily be adjusted for your weight loss goal and your nutritional needs. Keep the protein high and the carbohydrates low.

Sandwich #1, 107 calories, 10 grams of protein, 2 grams of fat, and 16 grams of carbohydrates. One slice low-calorie whole-wheat bread, one ounce of turkey breast, 1/8-ounce arugula lettuce, one tbsp. finely sliced sweet red pepper, and one tbsp. of mustard.

Sandwich #2, 136 calories, 10 grams of protein, 7 grams of fat, and 13 grams of carbohydrates. One slice of low-calorie whole-wheat bread, one ounce of sliced chicken breast, 1/8-ounce of celery leaf, and one tsp. of extra virgin olive oil.

Sandwich #3, 135 calories, 9 grams of protein, 7 grams of fat, and 13 grams of carbohydrates. One slice of low-calorie whole-wheat bread, one ounce of caned white tuna fish in water, one tbsp. minced onion, one tbsp. of diced celery, and one tbsp. of extra virgin olive oil.

Sandwich #4, 139 calories, 11 grams of protein, 6 grams of fat, and 12 grams of carbohydrates. One slice of low-calorie whole-wheat bread, one ounce of roast beef, one slice of tomato, and 1/8-tsp. of black pepper.

Sandwich #5, 183 calories, 13 grams of protein, 7 grams of fat, and 16 grams of carbohydrates. One slice of low-calorie whole-wheat bread, one ounce of swiss cheese, one slice of tomato, 1/8-ounce of arugula lettuce, and 1 tbsp. of mustard.

Sandwich #6, 148 calories, 6 grams of protein, 7 grams of fat, and 21 grams of carbohydrates. One slice of low-calorie whole-wheat bread, one ounce of canned, chopped chickpeas, one ounce of soy bean sprouts, one tsp. of sesame seed paste, and one tsp. of lemon juice.

Tortilla wrap #1, 93 calories, 11 grams of protein, 5 grams of fat, and 22 grams of carbohydrates. One low-calorie whole-wheat tortilla wrap, one ounce of sliced turkey breast, 2 tbsp. of diced cucumber, 1 tbsp. of diced jalapeno pepper, 1 tbsp. of sweet red pepper, and 1 tbsp. of sliced scallion.

Tortilla wrap #2, 104 calories, 11grams of protein, 4 grams of fat, and 21 grams of carbohydrates. One low-calorie whole-wheat tortilla wrap, one ounce sliced turkey breast, 1/8-ounce watercress lettuce, 2 tbsp. of sliced red onion, and one tbsp. of mustard.

Tortilla wrap #3, 123 calories, 14 grams of protein, 7 grams of fat, and 21 grams of carbohydrates. One low-calorie whole-wheat tortilla wrap, one ounce sliced chicken breast, 1/2-ounce diced avocado, 2 tbsp. diced tomato, 1 tbsp. onion, and 1 tbsp. lime juice.

Tortilla wrap #4, 179 calories, 9 grams of protein, 11 grams of fat, and 27 grams of carbohydrates. One low-fat whole-wheat tortilla wrap, one ounce canned and drained chopped chickpeas, 1 tbsp. diced red onion, 2 tbsp. sweet green pepper, and one tbsp. sesame seed paste.

Tortilla wrap #5, 136 calories, 8 grams of protein, 9 grams of fat, and 22 grams of carbohydrates. One low-fat whole-wheat tortilla wrap, two ounces of diced, firm tofu, 1/8-ounce of arugula lettuce, 1 tbsp. red onion, 1 tbsp. sweet red pepper, 1 tsp. extra virgin olive oil, and 1 tbsp. of lemon juice.

Tortilla wrap #6, 173 calories, 14 grams of protein, 8 grams of fat, and 21 grams of carbohydrates. One low-calorie whole-wheat tortilla wrap, one ounce of swiss cheese, 1/8-ounce of raw spinach, 2 tbsp. of red onion, and one tbsp. of mustard.

The following six recipes will all have this same procedure of assembly using three leafy lettuce leaves. Lay the leaves flat, long ways, and overlap by a third of a leaf. The ingredients will be laid on one end then rolled up. If you prefer, other varieties of lettuce can be used for the wraps.

Lettuce wrap #1, 136 calories, 12 grams of protein, 9 grams of fat, and 7 grams of carbohydrates. Three large red leafy lettuce leaves, 1 ounce of small cooked shrimp, 1/2-ounce finely sliced cabbage, 1 tbsp. diced sweet red pepper, 1 tsp. grated fresh ginger, 1 tbsp. sesame seed paste, and 1 tbsp. soy sauce.

Lettuce wrap #2, 90 calories, 11 grams of protein, 2 grams of fat, and 5 grams of carbohydrates. Three large red leafy lettuce leaves, 2 ounces of smoked salmon diced, 1/8-ounce shredded romaine lettuce, 1 tbsp. kalamata olives diced, 2 tbsp. red onion diced, and 2 tbsp. capers.

Lettuce wrap #3, 121 calories, 9 grams of protein, 8 grams of fat, and 4 grams of carbohydrates. Three large red leafy lettuce leaves, 1 ounce of sliced turkey breast, 1/2-strip cooked and diced bacon, 1/8-ounce shredded iceberg lettuce, one slice of tomato diced, 1 tsp. extra virgin olive oil, and 1 tbsp. balsamic vinegar.

Lettuce wrap #4, 137 calories, 4 grams of protein, 9 grams of fat, and 12 grams of carbohydrates. Three large red leafy lettuce leaves, 1 ounce of drained chickpeas chopped, 1/4-ounce sunflower seeds, 1/2-ounce fresh cilantro diced, 1/8-ounce iceberg lettuce shredded, 2 tbsp. red onion diced, 1 tsp. sesame seed oil, and 2 tbsp. lemon juice.

Lettuce wrap #5, 67 calories, 8 grams of protein, 3 grams of fat, and 8 grams of carbohydrates. Three large red leafy lettuce leaves, 1 ounce of chicken breast diced, 1/8-ounce of arugula lettuce, 2 tbsp. kalamata olives sliced, 1 tbsp. scallions diced, 1 tbsp. sweet red pepper diced, and 1 tbsp. red wine vinegar.

Lettuce wrap #6, 142 calories, 10 grams of protein, 6 grams of fat, and 10 grams of carbohydrates. Three large red leafy lettuce leaves, 1 ounce of sharp provolone diced, one slice of tomato diced, 2 tbsp. of dill pickle diced, 1 ounce of soy bean sprouts, 1 tbsp. of hot sauce, 1 tbsp. of balsamic vinegar, and 1 tbsp. of mustard.

Vegan/Vegetarian Hummus Variations

Simply choose one or several foods from categories A, B, C, D, and E. Either chop, slice, blend, or any way you choose to combine the ingredients. By choosing just one item from each of the three categories, A, B, and C, you will have a meal with complete proteins. You can use these hummus mixes in wraps, sandwiches, as dips, or as salad dressings.

Category A
Chickpeas-canned
Cooked lentils-red, yellow, or brown
Green pees
Soy beans
Beans-red, black, white, etc.

Category B
Corn-fresh or canned
Oats-cooked
Whole wheat-cooked
Brown rice-cooked
Wild rice-cooked
Quinoa-cooked
Buckwheat-cooked

<u>Category C</u>
Chia seeds
Sesame seeds
Sesame paste
Sunflower seeds
Pumpkin seeds
Hemp seeds
Walnuts
Hazelnuts
Pistachio nuts
Almonds
Pine nuts

<u>Category D</u>
Avocado
Sweet pepper
Hot pepper
Red or white onion
Scallion
Garlic
Tomato
Cucumber
Celery
Bean sprouts
Zucchini
Carrots
Beets

<u>Category E</u>
Lemon
Lime
Cilantro
Basil
Parsley
Oregano
Marjoram
Rosemary
Mint

Olive oil
Avocado oil
Coconut oil
Walnut oil
Peppermint oil

It can be challenging when you have very limited choices. Meals cooked without the addition of unnecessary fats and carbohydrates are your best choices. The methods of choice when you are having your food cooked are broiled, boiled, poached, steamed, baked, grilled, or microwaved. Stay away from fried foods, which have huge amounts of unwanted fat. Don't be compelled to have many courses of food or consume the same amount of food as your companions. It's okay to order one dish, one serving, or just have a drink!

The following are some choices you may want to consider when dining out.

Breakfast Choices

<u>Poached egg</u>, one whole egg, 71 calories, 6 grams of protein, 0 fat, 1 gram of carbohydrates.
<u>Poached egg whites</u>, 3 egg whites, 50 calories, 12 grams of protein, 0 fat, 1 gram of carbohydrates.
<u>Bacon,</u> 3 strips of cooked bacon, 109 calories, 6 grams of protein, 2 grams of fat, 0 carbohydrates.
<u>Grapefruit</u>, 1/2 grapefruit, 52 calories, 1 gram of protein, 0 fat, 13 grams of carbohydrates.

Lunch Choices

<u>Chicken, roasted</u>, 3 oz., 147 calories, 27 grams of protein, 3 grams of fat, 0 carbohydrates.
<u>Fish, baked</u>, 3oz., cod or other similar fish, 89 calories, 19 grams of protein, 1 gram of fat, 0 carbohydrates.
<u>Salad with 1 hardboiled egg</u>, 180 calories, 7 grams of protein, 1 gram of fat, 2 grams of carbohydrates.

Shrimp cocktail, 4 oz., 220 calories, 24 grams of protein, 4 grams of fat, 0 carbohydrates.

Hotdog on bun, 242 calories, 10 grams of protein, 15 grams of fat, 18 grams of carbohydrates.

Dinner Choices That are Readily Available

Chicken-breast, grilled, 6 oz., 294 calories, 54 grams of protein, 6 grams of fat, 0 carbohydrates.
Pork loin, broiled, 4 oz., 220 calories, 30 grams of protein, 11 grams of fat, 0 carbohydrates.
Lobster, broiled, 3 oz., 83 calories, 17 grams of protein, 1 gram of fat, 2 grams of carbohydrates.
NY strip steak, broiled, 4 oz., 219 calories, 33 grams of protein, 9 grams of fat, 0 carbohydrates.
Shrimp, broiled, 3 oz., 135 calories, 24 grams of protein, 2 gram of fat, 0 carbohydrates.

Italian Restaurant Choices

Salad with light dressing, 230 calories, 2 grams of protein, 5 grams of fat, 15 grams of carbohydrates.
Baked clams, 255 calories, 25 grams of protein, 7 grams of fat, 30 grams of carbohydrates.
Broccoli rabe, steamed, 6 oz., 56 calories, 6 grams of protein, 0 fat, 6 grams of carbohydrates.
Shrimp cocktail, 4 oz., 220 calories, 24 grams of protein, 4 grams of fat, 0 carbohydrates. Hotdog on bun, 242 calories, 10 grams of protein, 15 grams of fat, 18 grams of carbohydrates.
Flounder, broiled, 8 oz., 280 calories, 56 grams of protein, 4 grams of fat, 0 carbohydrates.
Braciola, 4 oz., 300 calories, 42 grams of protein, 12 grams of fat, 5 grams of carbohydrates.

Chinese Restaurant Choices

Salad with ginger dressing, 130 calories, 2 grams of protein, 1 gram of fat, 3 grams of carbohydrates.

Miso soup, 1 cup, 66 calories, 6 grams of protein, 3 grams of fat, 4 grams of carbohydrates.

Pork dumplings, 3 dumplings steamed, 130 calories, 15 grams of protein, 3 grams of fat, 15 grams of carbohydrates.

Tofu, braised, 3 oz., 180 calories, 15 grams of protein, 12 grams of fat, 22 grams of carbohydrates.

Steamed vegetables, 6 oz., 80 calories, 4 grams of protein, 2 grams of fat, 15 grams of carbohydrates.

Mahi-mahi, broiled, 4 oz., 192 calories, 18 grams of protein, 13 grams of fat, 1 gram of carbohydrates.

Lobster, broiled, 3 oz., 83 calories, 17 grams of protein, 1 gram of fat, 2 grams of carbohydrates.

Mexican Restaurant Choices

House salad with low calorie dressing, 230 calories, 2 grams of protein, 5 grams of fat, 15 grams of carbohydrates.

Avocado salad, small bowl, 290 calories, 31 grams of protein, 10 grams of fat, 24 grams of carbohydrates.

Black bean soup, 1 cup, 180 calories, 10 grams of protein, 2 grams of fat, 27 grams of carbohydrates.

Beef fajita, 1 fajita, 297 calories, 19 grams of protein, 13 grams of fat, 25 grams of carbohydrates.

Chicken taco, 1 taco, 185 calories, 13 grams of protein, 6 grams of fat, 19 grams of carbohydrates.

Fish tostada, 1 tostada, 190 calories, 17 grams of protein, 8 grams of fat, 13 grams of carbohydrates.

Pork burrito, 1 small pulled pork burrito, 296 calories, 23 grams of protein, 11 grams of fat, 35 grams of carbohydrates.

Seafood Restaurant Choices

Mussels, steamed, 3 oz., 147 calories, 20 grams of protein, 4 grams of fat, 6 grams of carbohydrates.

Clams, steamed, 20 small clams, 175 calories, 25 grams of protein, 2 grams of fat, 5 grams of carbohydrates.

Shrimp, grilled, 6 oz., 270 calories, 48 grams of protein, 4 gram of fat, 0 carbohydrates.

Oysters, raw, 6 oysters, 175 calories, 8 grams of protein, 11 gram of fat, 10 grams of carbohydrates.

Lobster, steamed, 6 oz., 170 calories, 34 grams of protein, 2 gram of fat, 5 grams of carbohydrates.

Tuna steak, grilled, 6 oz., 240 calories, 54 grams of protein, 2 gram of fat, 0 carbohydrates.

BBQ Restaurant Choices

Collard greens, boiled, 1 cup, 34 calories, 2 gram of protein, 0 fat, 8 grams of carbohydrates.

Corn on the cob, grilled,1 cob, 90 calories, 2 grams of protein, 0 fat, 14 grams of carbohydrates.

Biscuits-buttermilk, 3 biscuits, 150 calories, 4 grams of protein, 2 grams of fat, 29 grams of carbohydrates.

Baked beans, 6 oz., 267 calories, 15 grams of protein, 3 grams of fat, 47 grams of carbohydrates.

BBQ beef brisket, 3 oz., 280 calories, 32 grams of protein, 9 grams of fat, 25 grams of carbohydrates.

BBQ baby-back pork ribs, 3 ribs, 340 calories, 24 grams of protein, 23 grams of fat, 8 grams of carbohydrates.

Grilled chicken breast, 6oz, 294 calories, 54 grams of protein, 6 grams of fat, 0 carbohydrates.

Steakhouse Restaurant Choices

House salad with low calorie dressing, 230 calories, 2 grams of protein, 5 grams of fat, 15 grams of carbohydrates.

Shrimp cocktail, 4 oz., 220 calories, 24 grams of protein, 4 grams of fat, 0 carbohydrates.

Hotdog on bun, 242 calories, 10 grams of protein, 15 grams of fat, 18 grams of carbohydrates.

Broccoli, steamed, 3 oz., 30 calories, 2 grams of protein, 0 fat, 6 grams of carbohydrates.

French onion soup, with cheese, without the bread, 1 cup, 270 calories, 15 grams of protein, 19 grams of fat, 12 grams of carbohydrates.

Shrimp, grilled, 6 oz., 270 calories, 48 grams of protein, 4 grams of fat, 0 carbohydrates.

Pork loin, grilled, 4 oz., 220 calories, 30 grams of protein, 11 grams of fat, 0 carbohydrates.

NY strip steak, grilled, 4 oz., 219 calories, 33 grams of protein, 9 grams of fat, 0 carbohydrates.

Ribeye steak, grilled, 4 oz., 221 calories, 34 grams of protein, 9 grams of fat, 0 carbohydrates.

Lambchops, 4 oz., broiled, 222 calories, 17 grams of protein, 16 grams of fat, 0 carbohydrates.

Vegetarian Restaurant Choices

Hummus, served with vegetables, 4 oz., 220 calories, 8 grams of protein, 9 grams of fat, 17 grams of carbohydrates.

Grape leaves, stuffed with rice, 2 oz., 92 calories, 1 gram of protein, 3 grams of fat, 8 grams of carbohydrates.

Tofu, braised, 3 oz., 180 calories, 15 grams of protein, 12 grams of fat, 22 grams of carbohydrates.

Soybeans, steamed, 1/2 cup, cooked, 130 calories, 10 grams of protein, 5 grams of fat, 9 grams of carbohydrates.

Soybean sprouts, 1/2 cup, 40 calories, 5 grams of protein, 2 grams of fat, 2 grams of carbohydrates.

Lentil soup, 1 cup, 260 calories, 18 grams of protein, 3 grams of fat, 45 grams of carbohydrates.

Rice and beans, 1 cup, 220 calories, 7 grams of protein, 6 grams of fat, 36 grams of carbohydrates.

Dessert Choices

Coffee-plain, 8 oz., 2 calories, 0 protein, 0 fat, 0 carbohydrates.

Coffee-cappuccino, 8 oz., 77 calories, 4 grams of protein, 4 grams of fat, 6 grams of carbohydrates.

Coffee-espresso, 4 oz., 2 calories, 0 protein, 0 fat, 0 carbohydrates.

Blackberries-fresh, 1/2 cup, 31 calories, 1gram of protein, 0 fat, 7 grams of carbohydrates.

Blueberries-fresh, 1/2 cup, 41 calories, 1 gram of protein, 0 fat, 11 grams of carbohydrates.

Raspberries-fresh, 1 pt., 172 calories, 5 grams of protein, 1 gram of fat, 35 grams of carbohydrates.

<u>Strawberries-fresh</u>, 1 cup, 55 calories, 1 gram of protein, 0 fat, 10 grams of carbohydrates.

<u>Ice pop, 100% fruit juice</u>, 8 oz., 54 calories, 0 protein, 0 fat, 13 grams of carbohydrates.

<u>Honeydew-fresh</u>, 1 cup, 61 calories, 1 gram of protein, 0 fat, 15 grams of carbohydrates.

<u>Yogurt-plain</u>, whole milk, 8 oz., 140 calories, 7 grams of protein, 7 grams of fat, 12 grams of carbohydrates.

<u>Sherbet-orange</u>, 1/2 cup, 137 calories, 1 gram of protein, 1 gram of fat, 28 grams of carbohydrates.

<u>Crepes-plain</u>, 1 crepe, 112 calories, 4 grams of protein, 6 grams of fat, 11 grams of carbohydrates.

<u>Whipped cream</u>, 1 tbsp., 60 calories, 0 protein, 6 grams of fat, 6 grams of carbohydrates.

Chapter Three
Six Activities a Day

Why Six Activities a Day?

Activities take up time slots, keep your mind focused, burn calories, keep you energized, and enhance your life. The more strenuous activities will burn calories and build muscle mass, further accelerating your weight loss. Activities can also help achieve other goals besides weight loss.

You can create your activity program to focus on or achieve a specific goal, whether it's a hobby, a sport, an education program, or your unique objective. When your activities are systematically incorporated into Diet666, amazing rewards are to be had. Diet666 is a whole lifestyle program. Each aspect of this diet program is beneficial, but you will not get the tremendous results without implementing the program as a whole, all-encompassed diet concept.

Each of the high-protein meals will keep your body sustained for some time, it will vary with different individuals and different meal selections. The meals, while sustaining your body's needs, will also keep the hunger away. When the food is used up by the body the effects will dissipate, that's why the activities are needed. When done the right way, the hunger sensations throughout the day will be minimized. The hunger sensations will not be the type that will give you the feeling of starvation. By keeping yourself focused on the activities, it will keep your mind off the food.

The activities that work best are the ones that use both your body and your mind. The higher intensity activities work better at focusing both your body and your mind. When your body is being used at full capacity there is no hunger at all. When your mind is fully engulfed in thought there is no hunger. When you put the two together there is no room for hunger.

A person performing an intensive weightlifting workout will be using massive amounts of energy with no thoughts of hunger. When you have an intense chess game, you will have no feeling of hunger. When playing basketball, soccer, hokey, dancing, running, etc., there will be no hunger. Any and all activity help, whether it's reading an interesting book or skiing down black diamond trails.

Some activities are more beneficial than others in their own way. There are activities that keep your mind occupied and there are others that have the additional benefit of burning calories. All activities take up time slots and to varying extents they all keep hunger away. It's the consistency of six meals a day, six activities a day, six days a week, and a day of fasting that produces amazing results.

With the proper planning, you will have many activities of your choice available. When planning your activities consider your health and how intense your overall diet plan will be. Compile a list of activities that can easily be done then advance to the activities that are challenging at the appropriate time. Space the activities out in conjunction with the meals.

You can start your day either with a meal or an activity, then alternate throughout the rest of the day. It's better to alternate the meals and activities, but it doesn't always have to be that way. For instance, you may choose to have a morning meal, then go to the gym for an hour, then go to the library for an hour, and then have a meal. That would be meal, activity, activity, meal, then finish the day as usual, with a total of six meals and six activities.

The six meals and six activities a day for six days a week gives you the discipline that makes your mind and body strong. When Diet666 is working properly, your body will be deficient in calories every day. Because of this, your body will be accustomed to and very efficient at using your body's fat for energy. This will make you lose weight and will diminish your hunger. This is a major part of the plan, you will notice these effects after a week or two. Once in full swing, you will only get hints of hunger.

Types of Activities and Usefulness

There are thousands of activities available. Each of us have our own preferences and limitations. A medical doctor can help you set your limitations then you can compile an activity program that suits your goal.

During the course of this program you will most likely alter your program. You can alter your activity durations, change the types of activities, and change their intensities. The main thing is to do it, that is take up those time slots no matter what activity it is.

If you're tired, do a less exhausting activity. Be prepared for these moments. Have alternative activities, because things happen, don't use them for an excuse to fail. Always have a backup plan; do not under any circumstances give up. Whatever the obstacle may be—sickness, injury, friends, work, physically exhausted, or mentally drained—stay focused and stick with the plan.

Notice the plan calls for activities, not just exercises. This gives us a lot of options, from strenuous exercises to relaxing meditation, and everything in between. There are some activities that we don't count even though they do burn some calories, but by doing so would take up unnecessary time. These are things like seeing, hearing, thinking, breathing, eating, sleeping, listening to music, watching TV, or texting to name a few. I'm sure this list could go much further.

There will be enough calculating to be done tracking the consumption and the burning of calories without getting into every little aspect of it all. When we look at a day in anyone's life, there most likely will be activities. We can include our everyday activities into the overall plan.

There are some things we do on a regular basis. For instance, taking a shower, getting dressed, walking the dog/cat, shopping, cooking, cleaning, etc. Now here's the point, the main purpose of doing an activity is to take up some time so we don't count anything less than thirty minutes as one of the six activities. You can add up all the used calories for those five-minute things throughout the day and count them toward your burned daily calories, but don't count them as activities. I usually count all those little things as a total of 100 calories. I try not to get too petty with the tiny things. Don't count them as activities unless they are at least for a duration of half an hour, preferably longer. Activities that take an hour or more are best, they take up a nice piece of time and burn calories. If for some reason you do half an hour, that's all right, but your goal is to eventually reach an hour or longer.

Activities that are of consecutive hours count as one activity. This means that three hours in the gym, three hours cleaning your house, three hours of reading a book, or three hours performing your occupational work all count as one activity. This is how it's done, weight loss with little hunger.

You can easily change a three-hour activity if needed into something different. For example, instead of a three-hour gym activity counting as one activity, you could do one activity of one hour at the gym, then go to the library for an hour, which would be another activity. While at the library have a meal then go back to the gym for two hours. This would be activity (gym), meal, activity (library), then activity (gym). This is one example of the flexibility of combining activities and meals into your personal schedule.

After each meal wait a while before doing your next activity. This will give your body the time to start absorbing the nutrients of your meal and give you more time away from the sensations of hunger.

After each activity wait a while before having your next meal. This will help you relax and not be overly regimental. Activities can be classified in many ways. I will classify a few activities based on how hard they are to perform. We can usually take an activity and make it more or less intense to suit our goals. Notice that the plan calls for activities, which can be many types of things, including but not limited to exercises.

Easy Activities

This is a list of diversified activities and hobbies that are of low intensity. They will take time and will burn few calories unless performed for a long duration or more intensely.

Acting-either for fun as an amateur, working toward being a professional, or to improve your abilities
Animal interactions-caring for your pets, viewing them at a zoo or in their natural habitat
Aquarium-with either freshwater or saltwater fish
Astrology
Basket weaving or making gift baskets
Beach-sun tanning, walking, swimming
Beach-collecting shells
Beach-building sandcastles
Beadwork-create bracelets, necklaces, and works of art
Birdwatching and bird photography
Bonsai tree-collecting and maintaining
Bookbinding-put together your own book
Brewing beer-create your own micro-brewery
Building dollhouses-design and create your very own
Butterfly watching and photography
Calligraphy-express your handwriting
Candle making
Cartoon drawing
Casino gambling
Ceramics
Charity work-for people, animals, or the environment; this can be rewarding in many ways
Church-prayers or other spiritual activities
Collecting-coins, guitars, baseball cards, dolls, rocks, antiques, etc.
Coloring books-it's fun and not just for kids
Computer activities-the possibilities are endless
Cooking as a hobby-not for an excuse to overeat!
Crocheting
Darts-alone, with a friend, or on a team

Digital photography-there are many areas in this field to explore
Embroidery
Fishing
Floral arrangements
Games-board or video
Gardening-create your magic garden
Ghost hunting
Glass-making, blowing, etching, beadmaking, stained glass
Go to the movies
Guitar or other instrument-playing
Horse-riding or grooming
Hot air ballooning
Inventing
Jewelry-making or repairing
Juggling
Kite flying-kites come in a variety of shapes and sizes
Knitting
Learning and education
Learning a foreign language or sign language
Learning to play different types of instruments
Leather crafting
Magic-be a magician
Marksmanship-target shooting or skeet shooting
Meditation
Metal detecting-looking for valuable metal on land or sea
model cars-building them from a kit
Model railroads-with trains and miniature landscapes
Model rockets-fun for all ages
Model ship building
Mosaics
Paper making-paper mâché, paper sculpture
Photography-film or digital, B&W, color, people, pets, underwater,
etc.
Playing music-listening
Puzzles-crossword or jigsaw
Quilting
Racing pigeons

Reading-at a library, bookstore, or home, cyber or not
Remote control-boats, cars, drones, helicopters, planes, etc.
Rescuing-helping animals that are abused or abandoned
Robotics-create and control miniature robots
Scrapbook-create your own personal scrapbook
Sculpture-numerous techniques, using various types of materials such as paper, wax, clay, wood, metal, plastic, glass, etc.
Sewing-create your own clothing line or maybe just do some patchwork
Shopping-America's favorite pastime
Soap making-experiment with different additives
Socializing-in person, by phone, texting, social media, etc.
Spending time entertaining family and friends
Stretching as a low-intensity activity, a relaxing stretch
Treasure hunting-by land, sea, internet, pawnshops, or flea markets
TV watching-an easy way to use large amounts of time
Watching sports and other events-either at a stadium, arena, a stage, or on TV
Woodworking projects
Working on cars, motorcycles or bicycles
Yoga-at a low intensity
Writing-fiction, nonfiction, music, songs, poetry, etc.

Moderate Activities

Keep in mind most activities can be performed at different levels of intensity.

Acrobatics
Badminton
Baseball
Basketball
Bicycling
Boating-operating a sailboat
Bodybuilding
Bowling
Camping and hiking
Canoeing

Cliff diving
Fencing
Football
Hang gliding
Ice skating
Jumping rope
Kayaking
Kite boarding
Martial arts-jujitsu, mixed martial arts, boxing, etc.
Paintball
Paragliding
Playing various types of unmentioned sports
Rafting
Rollerblading
Scuba diving
Sky diving
Snorkeling
Snowboarding
Snow skiing or water skiing
Soccer
Surfing
Survival training
Swimming
Tennis
Various types of gym machines
Walking-briskly or walking up hills
Weightlifting
Windsurfing
Yoga
Zumba

Intense, Very Intense, or Extreme Activities

Many activities, including the list of easy and moderate activities, can be brought up a few notches by performing them faster, harder, and/or longer. The following is a list of activities that I recommend for intense, very intense, or extreme activities, considering you are at that level of fitness. Don't advance too fast and never go beyond your ability.

Acrobatics
Base jumping
Basketball
Bicycling
Bodybuilding
Bull riding
Cliff diving
Dancing
Football
Frisbee
Gymnastics
Gym workouts
Handball
Hiking
Hockey
Ice skating
Jumping rope
Kiteboarding
Lacrosse
Motocross
Mountain climbing
Occupations-masonry, carpentry, iron worker, tree trimming, etc.
Paddleboarding
Rafting
Rock climbing
Rollerblading
Rugby
Running-fast, hills, sprints, marathons, etc.
Sailboat-operating
Self-defense-boxing, mixed martial arts, karate, judo, etc.
Skateboarding
Skiing-snow or water
Snowboarding
Soccer

Surfing
Survival training
Swimming
Tennis and table tennis
Triathlon
Volleyball
Wakeboarding
Water polo
Weightlifting
Wind surfing
Wrestling

The planning of your activities starts by knowing the amount of time you're dealing with. Consider your daily personal responsibilities, which may be your household chores, your occupation, education, etc. Decide on the segments of time that you will choose for your activities. Keep in mind that everyone will design their own unique diet plan and can alter it as needed.

Let's start with an example of how a person might deal with the 24-hour day. For this example, the day of fasting is not included because it has its own set of procedures.

First, we start with the 24-hour day then we take away eight hours that are used for sleeping. We now have sixteen hours left in which we will consume our meals, perform our activities, and everything else we do in life.

We now look at all of our responsibilities, the things that need to be done, not including the diet plan. Some of these things you may decide to count as activities and incorporate them into your activity plan. For instance, if you spend some time at work (1/2 hr., 1 hr., 2 hrs.) performing a physically strenuous or mind-intense job, you can surely count this as one of your activities. Set your activities schedule in conjunction with or around your daily responsibilities.

After this, consider when you will be having your meals. There are times when you will need to work around certain meals that are not part of your diet plan, such as dinner engagements, parties, and social events. Keep some time between the activities and the meals, don't rush. Try to alternate between meals and activities. The meals usually take a short time and can easily be had. The activities, on the other hand, are much longer. If you wanted, you could do six activities of two and a half hours each. This would be a total of fifteen hours and would use the whole day, leaving you with only time for your six meals and little time for hunger!

For those people who have personal responsibilities that change from day to day, hour to hour, your activities can be altered or totally changed to conform to a changing schedule. When something interrupts your plan, just pick up from where you left off. Try your hardest to make this plan your priority, don't let unnecessary things get in your way.

If you are sick, injured, or have a disability, take this into account when choosing your activities. Activities can be something that you enjoy and look forward to, not just time consuming. You can structure your activities toward a specific goal. This will be much more rewarding by adding to the benefits of your weight loss. Use your imagination, get thin while working toward a goal.

The basics of getting a plan started is to know your limitations. Consider your basic sleep patterns and plan your day with six meals and six activities included. Plan around or in conjunction with your daily commitments. Plan reasonable activities considering your physical and mental abilities. You will add and increase calorie burning activities when possible, alter your plan as needed, be consistent with six meals a day, six activities a day, and doing this for six days a week then fasting.

I created lists of activities for you to choose from but don't be confused, you don't need an extensive amount of activities. You can simply use one or a few activities and increase their intensity. For example, if walking is the only activity that's going to be used for all of your six activities, you can simply increase the intensity by extending the duration then walk faster and add up-hill trails.

Here is a simple schedule to demonstrate the timing of the six activities and six meals. Try to have a meal after every activity. This is the ideal situation but not absolutely necessary. In practicality, the times of the meals and activities will be decided when you create your own personal plan. You decide on the timing, whatever works best for yourself.

<u>Sleep</u>	12 a.m. to 8 a.m.
<u>Activity 1</u>, gym	9 a.m. to 10:45 a.m.
<u>Meal 1</u>, turkey wrap	10:45 a.m. to 11 a.m.
<u>Activity 2</u>, read a book	11:15 a.m. to 12:15 p.m.
<u>Meal 2</u>, beef jerky	12:30 p.m. to 12:45 p.m.
<u>Activity 3</u>, play the guitar	1 p.m. to 2 p.m.
<u>Meal 3</u>, shrimp wrap	2 p.m. to 2:15 p.m.
<u>Activity 4</u>, outdoor photography	2:30 p.m. to 4:30 p.m.
<u>Meal 4</u>, grilled fish	5 p.m. to 5:15 p.m.
<u>Activity 5</u>, shopping	5:30 p.m. to 7:30 p.m.
<u>Meal 5</u>, chicken sandwich	7:4 5p.m. to 8 p.m.
<u>Activity 6</u>, yoga	8:15 p.m. to 9:15 p.m.
<u>Meal 6</u>, turkey wrap	9:15 p.m. to 9:30 p.m.

The following activities are estimates of the calories used by a 200 lb. person in the course of an hour. This will vary depending on the person's weight, metabolism, and the intensity level of performance. You can use these estimates to calculate similar activities.

Aerobics 465
Basketball 550
Bicycling-fast 900
Bicycling-slow 370
Billiards 230
Bird watching 250
Boating 230
Bowling 280
Calisthenics 432
Carpentry 350
Cleaning the house 300
Dancing 300

Driving-car 90

Driving-motorcycle 160

Drum playing 260

Football 700

Frisbee 380

Gardening 320

Golfing 420

Gymnastics 370

Handball 1000

Hiking 550

Hockey 745

Horseback riding 326

Ice skating 512

Jogging four miles an hour 600

Jumping rope 745

Kayaking 465

Laughing 120

Martial arts/boxing 931

Meditation 75

Mowing lawn/walking 512

Paddleboard 558

Painting 419

Piano playing 150

Playing with children 260

Pushing stroller with child 233

Pushing wheelchair 372

Reading 90

Rollerblading 651

Running at a pace of five miles an hour 745

Scuba diving 400

Shoveling snow or dirt 558

Singing 140

Skateboarding 465

Skiing-downhill 465

Skiing-water 558

Snorkeling 465

Softball 465

Stretching-mild 233
Surfing 350
Swimming-leisurely 558
Table tennis 372
Tennis 651
Vacuuming-house, car, etc. 200
Volleyball 745
Walking-slow 270
Walking with dog 320
Water aerobics 372
Weightlifting 400
Windsurfing 333
Writing 80

Chapter Four
Fasting

The Benefits of Fasting

Fasting is a key component of Diet666. The primary benefits are losing calories, resting your body's digestive system, resting your body's muscles, and focusing your mind. The simple aspect is that by not eating for the day you are calorie deficient, meaning weight loss is taking place. By being calorie deficient, your body uses stored fat for energy. When being calorie deficient every single day, your body gets increasingly better at using the stored body fat for energy. This is one of the great benefits that is built into the Diet666 weight loss program. This is a great help during your fast, you may find yourself totally without hunger for the whole day.

Your body is being trained to control hunger at a metabolic level, not just by meals, activities, and willpower. The fast gives your mind and body a break from your daily routine. Your body will get a chance to recuperate from strenuous exercises, if you're at that level of training. The fast can be a day of reflection, meditation, religious prayer, light activities, hobbies, etc. Perhaps you could save that special project that's on your to-do list for this special day. On this day, you will be enjoying the great feeling of success and self-accomplishment. Just think, you will have completed a full week of your Diet666 and tomorrow is the day to check your weight. The reward for your dedication is waiting. Checking your weight takes place only once a week, that is the day after the fast, which is also the morning of the first day of your new week.

How to Fast

For the purpose of this Diet666 weight loss plan, the fast takes place once a week on the last day of the week. You choose on which day of the week your dieting plan will start on, whatever is convenient for yourself. Previously, you have had six meals a day and performed six activities a day for six consecutive days. Ideally, each day your calorie count was deficient, meaning that for all of those six days your body needed to use your stored body fat for energy. Your body will not be shocked by fasting because it is now well prepared for the process of using your stored fat for energy.

To make the transition into the day of fasting easy, on the day before the fast have fewer than usual of your total calories for that day. It's much easier to go from low calories to no calories than from high calories to no calories. The consumption on the fasting day is basically zero calories. Have your normal sleep but don't sleep the day away. That's not necessary. Start the day with a multivitamin and a drink. All day long you will be having drinks that contain zero calories. Be sure to have many varieties of these drinks available. A few suggestions for your drinks are: water, flavored sparkling water, soft drinks without calories, some zero-calorie caffeinated soft drinks, iced tea, hot tea, hot coffee, and iced coffee.

If you're going to drink coffee or tea, avoid adding milk and don't add sugar. Coffee has a few calories in it, this is allowed because of the benefit that caffeine has on suppressing your appetite. Don't have caffeinated drinks within four hours of your bedtime, you don't want to stay awake unnecessarily. You can easily do this fast with no caffeine at all, it's your choice. Too much caffeine will give you up and down mood swings, try not to depend on the caffeine.

Be prepared for the day, have your supplies of liquids available. Have a list of light activities available to be used as you see fit. Physically, the previous days prepared you for your fast, now it's all about having a mental strategy. Being bored is your worst enemy, when this happens it's activity time.

Have a plan. Here are a few ways to handle a severe hunger urge. Try not to let it get this far, hunger will gradually creep up on you. Have a drink either ice cold or hot. Suck on a piece of ice or a zero-calorie ice pop, have a caffeinated drink or two, get out of the house and go for a walk or jog, go for a swim, do some type of activity. Take a shower; an ice-cold shower will destroy hunger. Take a nap. Have a coach available to talk to. You can put a few of these things together. For example, have a caffeinated drink, take the ice-cold shower, then go for a jog.

Keeping a journal can be a useful tool for your future fasts. Take notes of your feelings, activities, drinks, sleeping duration, and your time schedule for the day.

Activities During the Fast

Choosing your activities in advance is a good starting point, but while fasting things may change. It's perfectly fine if you choose to alter your day to suit your needs. For instance, if you planned on staying home and playing the guitar all day but you got the urge to go to the beach, just do it!

Now for the activity suggestions. These are only a few low-intensity activities: arts and crafts projects; bicycle riding; boat ride; concert; fishing; fix those things around the house; fly a kite or drone; play games, either board or video; hobbies; house cleaning; kayaking; listening to music; make something; meditate; miniature golf; motorcycle ride; movies; play an instrument; do puzzles, either crossword or jigsaw; reading; go to a show or event; snorkeling; do something new; do a special project; swimming; walking around the block, park, beach, or trail; writing a poem, music, journal, or book.

Your own personal activities are what will make this work. For the first few times that you fast, use non-exhausting activities. This will keep your body from going into a severe hunger mode. After a few times fasting you may use a more intense but not exhausting activity, something like a slow jog. You may choose something new in your life and do it only on your fasting day. If you are performing at the Diet666 extreme level, you will be using some intense, high-calorie-burning activities.

Plan Your Day

The previous six days prepared your body's metabolism for the fast. You have created a list of activities that you will be using. You have all your liquids available. Now it's time to set a flexible schedule for the fast. You can alter your schedule as the day progresses, but you should have a starting plan.

Your fast starts after your last meal on your sixth day, and it ends on the first day of your new week. Remember, you choose the starting day of your plan, you don't have to start your Diet666 week on a Sunday.

Here is an example of the ideal fasting duration. Your fast starts on day six, which happens to be a Sunday, and your last meal takes place at eight p.m. You will be fasting from eight p.m. on Sunday through Monday, then end your fast by having your first meal at eleven a.m. on Tuesday. Tuesday will be your first day of your new Diet666 week. The fast would have been for thirty-nine hours. Performed in this time sequence, your following week will be easy to transition into.

A large portion of the thirty-nine hours is sleep. Sleeping from eleven p.m. on Sunday to nine a.m. on Monday is ten hours. Sleeping from eleven p.m. on Monday to nine a.m. on Tuesday is ten hours. This is a total of twenty sleeping hours. This is just an example, I don't always sleep ten hours!

There will be a few awake hours before sleeping on Sunday and a few awake hours on Tuesday. On Monday, there are primarily fourteen hours to concentrate on. This is just a broad outline, everyone will customize their own unique plan.

Here's a simple plan of activities for the fourteen hours. From nine a.m. to ten a.m., wake up, take a shower, get dressed, have a multivitamin, and drink a water. From ten a.m. to twelve p.m., have a coffee, take care of the pool, yard, plants, trees, and the house to-do list. From twelve p.m. to three p.m., hang out at the beach, swim, stroll, relax, and have a few waters. From three p.m. to five p.m., go to the park for a walk, then sit at a bench and read a book. From five p.m. to seven p.m., do an arts and crafts project. From seven p.m. to ten p.m., go to the movies. From ten p.m. to the time you go to sleep, watch TV in bed as you fall asleep. Have plenty of zero-calorie drinks throughout the day. Don't have caffeinated drinks close to bedtime.

Why is Fasting Not so Hard?

The fundamental, underlining reason why fasting isn't hard is because us humans are designed to fast. We fast every day when we sleep, then we typically break the fast by having a break-fast. Our ancestors, who existed thousands of years ago, went for long periods of time without food. For thousands of years, our ancestors did not have the capabilities to have food readily available on a daily basis.

We now live in an environment where we have food so readily available that our bodies seldom use the process of using our stored fat for energy. We are accustomed to storing fat on our bodies and not using it. Our ancestors, unlike us, went without food for lengths of time on a regular basis. When there was food, they ate, when there wasn't food, they didn't. Their bodies were accustomed to using their stored body fat for energy.

Being calorie deficient each and every day will get your body accustomed to using your body fat for energy, just as our ancestors did on a regular basis. This will reduce hunger and fatigue, making every day with low or no calorie consumption easy. This is an amazing process that your body and mind will adjust to. Our bodies' built-in process of using fat for energy is incorporated into this Diet666 program.

Planning the day for your sleeping times, liquids, and activities will make the day go smoothly. Having a strong determination to succeed will get you by any difficulties. By having read and fully understanding this book, you will make wise decisions. Before your fasting day, you will have already completed the six days of six meals and six activities and feeling proud of yourself. You are looking forward to the next day standing on the scale looking down and being amazed at all the weight you lost. Get past the fast and start your next week as a lighter you!

Alternatives

The optimal starting point for fasting is when you are losing weight every day. On the sixth day, you should have lower calorie consumption compared to the previous five days. Don't eat more the day before the fast, thinking that the extra food will be an asset. It will work against you by making you hungry. Less is best. If you are not at the point of doing a full fast, there are other options available until you get there.

Instead of fasting on day seven, you could do a few non-strenuous activities and have a few low-calorie meals. You can have no activities at all and have just a few meals. On day seven, you can simply have less calories than the day before with or without activities. Do not have a large number of calories on this day. If you do, it will be harder for you on the following days.

You can start training for your fast by doing a mini fast, waiting five, ten, or fifteen hours before your first meal. Remember, this diet plan has many aspects to it and fasting on the seventh day is an important one. Whether you fast on the first week or if it takes you a few weeks, it's fine as long as you get there. The diet is six meals and six activities for six days then fast.

Further Benefits of Fasting

There are claims that fasting has many benefits besides the ones I outlined for the purpose of this book. As far as I can determine, the following are possible benefits, not definite ones. They are not thoroughly researched but are still worth mentioning.

–Fasting may slow down aging
–Prolong life expectancy
–Have a positive impact on diabetics
–Have a positive effect on cardiovascular disease
–Help with atherosclerosis, high blood pressure, and high cholesterol

–Help with arthritis, joint pain, and osteoporosis
–Reboot the hormones and genes in the body
–Can boost the body's human growth hormone
–Help the process of cell repair
–Reduce inflammation and oxidation stress in the body
–Increase the quality of a person's skin
–Help with acne, eczema, psoriasis, and wrinkles
–Strengthen the immune system
–Help repair various types of brain injuries
–Slow down the decline in a person's mental ability
–Lesson the effects of Alzheimer's disease
–Help with anxiety, tension, depression, and fatigue
–May have positive effects on cancer
–Build self-control, self-confidence, and character

Fasting: The Dos and Don'ts

Do plan which day of the week that you will be fasting on.
Do plan out your whole day of fasting.
Do get plenty of sleep the night before your fast.
Do drink lots of liquids during your fast.
Don't do a full fast until you're totally ready for it, body and mind.
Don't overeat the day before the fast. Eat less, not more.
Don't choose the day of fasting that's not convenient.
Don't consume calories when fasting, by either food or liquid.
Don't consume caffeinated drinks close to bedtime.

We fast way more than you might think. Whether it's unintentional or intentional, we all skip meals at one time or another, this is kind of a mini fast. When we sleep, we fast for many hours. When we get sick, we sometimes fast, it's part of our natural healing process.

Chapter Five
Planning Options

Planning for Different Situations

There are many aspects in life that must be considered when configuring your own Diet666 program. I will present a few scenarios that you can examine and then modify for your personal goals.

The first is for a person that doesn't have a job, has no mandatory responsibilities, and has nothing that will interfere with any aspect of their diet plan. Basically, in this scenario, any day of the week can be used for fasting, and any time schedule for the meals and the activities will be fine. This is the ideal situation.

The second is for a person that has a steady work schedule, perhaps a nine to five job with weekends off. In this scenario, it would be wise to first choose the fasting day, perhaps Sunday. The next consideration is your activities. Will your work performance suffice as an activity, or two, or three, etc.? Choose the six activities that you will use for the day. Determine what meals you will have and when you will have them. For instance, if you're a carpenter that does four two-hour jobs a day, this can be counted as four activities. Take a break between jobs to have a meal. If it's a nine to five job, sitting at a desk and answering phones a few times a day, this can be counted as one activity.

The third is a person that has various responsibilities, commitments, and goals. This is the time to prioritize and organize the schedule for your six meals and activities, six days a week. Choose a convenient day for your fasting. There may be a need to change the timing of your personal responsibilities.

The fourth is for when there are special considerations. There can be conditions like mental or physical disabilities. There can also be spiritual or psychological concerns. A personal or medically restrictive diet may be required. Perhaps a person with severe obesity needs special attention. In these instances, constant supervision by a medical professional may be needed. Carefully consider the meals, activities, and whether or not fasting is appropriate. When a person has severe or compound complications, it's best to gradually work into a dieting program. Going slow and steady in these cases is the best method. Over time, the health complications may improve, and at that point, a more intense Diet666 program can be considered.

Adding Sports Training to the Program

For a more rewarding and interesting program, there can be specific goals added, such as incorporating sports training. The best way to add sports training to the program is to first discuss your intentions with a medical doctor, ensuring you're capable and fit enough to proceed without any adverse effects. Follow the basic plan for a few weeks and then include the activities specifically designed to enhance the sport of your choice. You can swap out a few of your usual activities for a few activities that are chosen for your sport of choice.

When you're ready, you can use all of your six activities to focus specifically on your chosen sport. Ensure you have the proper sleep and stay hydrated. Design your meals considering the activities you will be performing. Your meals may need more protein and carbohydrates than usual to support the intensity of your activities.

Since I can't account for the training programs of every sport, I will give you a few ideas that can be adjusted to fit many types of sports. Depending on your goals, you can adjust the activities to fit your needs.

Some low-intensity activities for learning the sport can be watching the sport being played, either live or on video, reading related books, or listening to live or recorded audio. Intense activities can be exercises at the gym specific to the sport, doing the sport under the supervision of a personal trainer, having a class with group lessons, doing the sport with a few friends, performing the sport with a team, or doing outside and inside training.

For instance, if the chosen sport is tennis, a six-activity day may be something like this. Activity one, reading a book about the rules and methods of tennis. Activity two, outdoor running with sprints. Activity three, aerobics specific for tennis performed at the gym. Activity four, watch a video of tennis matches or tennis techniques. Activity five, be instructed by a professional trainer. Activity six, play with a friend or team.

Use your own specific time to perform each activity and set the durations of your activities. Everyone needs to plan their own schedule, knowing their own unique capabilities and starting point.

Adding Hobbies: Music, Art, Education, etc.

There are basic similarities to adding hobbies as with adding sports activities. Hobbies and similar activities are usually less strenuous then most sports activities. Hobbies and similar activities will focus your mind, burn some calories, take up some of your time, keep hunger away, add enjoyment, and boost your feelings of self-accomplishment.

You can easily incorporate any type of hobby or educational program while implementing your diet plan. Because hobbies typically don't use massive amounts of calories, your typical meal plan will suffice. You may or may not need to increase your protein and daily calorie count, depending on the intensity levels of your activities. Your specific activities and meals will be planned around your unchangeable daily responsibilities. You can use your activity plan as a path toward becoming a skilled artesian or a professional of your choice. Plan your goals and acknowledge your accomplishments. Swap activities in and out of your plan as you see fit. Keep it fun while losing weight!

Here is an example of the Diet666 plan that includes a special hobby, which is learning to do drawings. First, define the preliminary schedule with the times of your personal responsibilities along with the meals and activities. The activities will focus on the art of drawing. The next step is to gather your supplies. Drawing supplies could include paper pads, black and colored pencils, eraser, pens, charcoal, instruction books, videos, and other reference material.

A day of six activities may be something like this: Activity one, read an instruction book on the methods of drawing for two hours. Activity two, using your instruction book, do a simple drawing using charcoal for an hour. Activity three, view art at a museum for two hours. Activity four, at an art studio receive personal instruction for an hour. Activity five, practice at home what was learned from your personal instruction. Activity six, do some experimental drawings using a variety of methods for an hour.

When learning any hobby there are a few points that should be considered—the style, instruction, and implementation. Determining your style may take some time. Examine the different aspects of your hobby then experiment with them. The instruction can be from a person, book, or video. The implementation is practice, practice, practice. You can join a club, school, or group specific to the hobby of your choice. A friend with mutual interests may be your hobby partner.

Intensity of Weight Loss

When choosing the intensity of your Diet666 program, first consider your physical and mental ability with the supervision of a medical doctor. Determine your starting weight and your goal weight. Decide how fast you want to lose the weight. The more intense programs will produce faster weight loss, requiring more diligence and determination. Consider what in your life you are willing to change or do without in order to reach your goal. Know what is reasonable for yourself after considering your health, determination, goals, and every aspect of your life.

It may be easier to start with a low-intensive plan for the first week. This will help you adjust your life in conjunction with your meals, activities, and fasting schedule. Strive to get on a daily and weekly schedule, this will give your body and mind stability.

I will outline a few basic plans with varying intensities. In reality, the variations are endless. The goal of these varying plans is to give you some insight into the versatility of Diet666. You can use any one of these plans and alter it for your own personal needs. Keep in mind that there are variations of weight loss due to water retention, muscle mass, height, age, gender, metabolism, and a person's weight variations. As your weight decreases, so does your basic daily calorie needs. This means a 200 lb. person needs 2,000 calories to sustain their weight for the day. For a 190 lb. person, it's 1,900 calories; for a 180 lb. person, it's 1,800 calories, etc.

For simplicity, the following examples are for a 200 lb. person.

The very-low-intensity program is designed for the person who wants to start slow by getting the fundamentals of Diet666 correct and then going with a more intense program. For this type of plan the weight loss goal is between a half-pound and one pound per week.

Determine what your starting calorie count is for a day. The simple way to estimate this is by multiplying your weight by ten. If for example you are 200 lbs., you would multiply this by ten, giving you 2,000 calories. This means you use 2,000 calories through the day by just existing, using only basic body functions. Keep in mind as you lose weight you are also changing your daily starting calorie count. The more weight you lose, the less calories are needed to sustain your body.

This very-low-intensity plan calls for six meals a day for either six or seven days. The total calories consumed each day will be ten percent less than your daily starting calories. For this example, 2,000 calories less ten percent is 1,800 calories. Now, by dividing the 1,800 calories by six meals, you will have six meals that consist of

300 calories each. Prepare the meals so that they are high in protein, low in fat, and low in carbohydrates.

Do six non-strenuous activities, paced throughout the day. On day seven, try to do a mini fast of six, eight, ten, or twelve hours. Either have six meals or eliminate some of them. Depending on the fasting and the chosen activities, this would bring a weight loss of between a half-pound and a full pound for the week. For example, 200 fewer calories a day, less 100 calories a day for basic daily activities, such as cleaning, cooking, household chores, etc., and burning 100 calories a day from the six light activities. The total deduction of your daily calories is 400. Multiply this by seven days and you get a loss of 2,800 calories for the week. Close to 3,500 calories, which would be a pound.

There can be a much larger weight loss due to a reduction of salt in your diet. By drastically reducing salt and salt products, you can lose a huge amount of weight. This is basically a one-time deal. If you return to consuming moderate amounts of salt, the water weight you lost will inevitably return.

I will give you an example of a very-low-intensity program. Keep in mind, this is for you to use as reference, you will form your own personal diet plan.

First, make sure you are medically and physically fit before proceeding. Decide on the day you will start and the times you will be having the meals and performing the activities. You weigh yourself once a week on the morning of the first day of your week. Each of the six meals will have 300 calories and be high in protein. No sugar. An example of this type of meal can be a sandwich consisting of two slices of low-calorie whole-wheat bread, four ounces of turkey breast, one slice of tomato, lettuce, a slice of onion, and a teaspoon of mustard. This is approximately 300 calories, thirty-two grams of protein, seven grams of fat, and thirty grams of carbohydrates. At this level, sugar and sugar products are eliminated but carbohydrates are not drastically reduced.

Use similar calorie and nutrient contents for all of your meals throughout the week. Alter the meals for your own preference focusing on the nutrition fundamentals.

The activities for the week will be of low intensity. For example, activities one, two, and three can be a slow walk for twenty minutes, each time burning about 100 total calories. If it's not possible for you to walk, try to do three other activities to burn the 100 calories. Activities four, five, and six can be reading a book for an hour, going shopping for an hour, and going to the movies for two hours. Do six activities, whatever you choose is fine. The important part is to do six activities. For this level, keep the activities at a low intensity. Day seven is the day of fasting. Do a mini fast waiting six, eight, or ten hours between your meals and activities. The meals and activities should be similar to the previous six days, but you can have fewer meals.

The low-intensity program is another great place to start. It's not shockingly intense and will focus on the fundamentals of the overall Diet666 program of six meals, six activities, for six days and fasting. This program takes a little more effort but is still a gradual transition toward major weight loss. This plan differs from the previous plan with changes in meals, activities, and fasting.

For a 200 lb. person, the basic formula is 200 multiplied by ten, which equals 2,000 calories. This is the starting calorie count that's needed for the daily body functions. The daily calorie reduction from meals will be by twenty percent. This formula is by starting with 2,000 calories less twenty percent (400 calories), which equals 1,600 calories. The daily calorie consumption will be 1,600. This is divided by six. Each meal for the day will be about 266 calories. The six activities used will be strenuous enough to burn twenty percent of your starting calorie count. Twenty percent of 2,000 is 400.

I suggest when starting at this level use four separate activities that burn 100 calories each and do two activities that burn very little calories. Alternatively, this can be done with two moderate calorie burning activities, burning 200 calories for each, and four low calorie burning activities. You might choose to do only one activity that burns 400 calories and five other low-intensity activities. Burn the 400 calories any way you want using the six daily activities. On the seventh day, the fasting will be of twelve, eighteen, or twenty-four hours. Do the fast between your six meals. You may choose to have fewer than six meals. Continue with consuming 1,600 calories for the day. There will be no or little activity on this day.

The total weight loss for the week will be about one and a half pounds. This may not sound like much, but if done for twenty weeks, you would have lost a total of thirty pounds. Choosing your options, preparing the meals, and selecting your activities is the fun part. You are creating your very own Diet666 program that will enhance your life. Design the plan for your personal needs.

These plans are guides, rough outlines for you to alter. Here is an example of this low-intensity plan. The meal is a chicken sandwich consisting of two slices of low-calorie whole-wheat bread, three ounces of chicken breast, two slices of tomato, one slice of onion, one ounce of sliced mushrooms, and a teaspoon of balsamic vinegar. This is about 262 calories, twenty-seven grams of protein, six grams of fat, and thirty-five grams of complex carbohydrates. Use similar meals six times a day for the week.

You will be burning about 400 calories a day by using some low-intensity activities along with your other non-intensive activities. For example, for the four low-intensity fat burning activities, do two twenty-minute walks, twenty minutes of stretching exercises, and then ride a bicycle for twenty minutes. For the other two activities, read a book for an hour then do a hobby of your choice for an hour. On day seven, have six meals similar to the previous day. Do little or no activities. Fast for twelve, eighteen, or twenty-four hours in-between your meals.

It would be something like this: Meal one, meal two, meal three, fast for twelve hours, meal four, meal five, then meal six. You select the timing. You can choose to have fewer than six meals on this day of fasting.

The medium-intensity program is where significant weight loss takes place in a shorter time frame. It is similar to the previous plans but more intense. The 200 lb. person starts with the calorie count of 2,000. This plan is a reduction of thirty percent, which will be 600 from the 2,000. That is 1,400 calories for the day. This will be six meals a day of 233 calories each.

Design your activity program so that it burns 600 calories a day and includes a total of six activities. Day seven is a full fast of twenty-four, thirty, or thirty-six hours. The goal is to have zero calories throughout the fast. There will be little or no activities for this day. If this type of Diet666 program is performed for ten weeks, there will be approximately twenty-five pounds lost.

An example of a meal at this level is one low-calorie tortilla wrap with two ounces of turkey, one ounce of low-fat cheese, and one sliced dill pickle. This is about 233 calories, twenty-four grams of protein, nine grams of fat, and twenty-one grams of carbohydrates. Use meals of similar nutrition and calorie content.

An activity example for a day at this level is a one-hour walk that burns 200 calories, half an hour doing yoga burning 100 calories, and one hour at the gym burning 300 calories. For non-intensive activities it can be shopping for an hour, doing household chores for an hour, and doing a crossword puzzle for an hour. Use activities of your choice to accomplish these goals.

The high-intensity program is similar to the previous programs with a few changes. At this level it's critical to be mentally and physical capable to proceed. This plan is very calorie restrictive and physically exerting. At this level of limited daily calories, it can be challenging to maintain a complete, nutritious diet. When considering your meals, keep in mind the nutritional aspects along with the diminished calories. Take nutritional supplements as needed.

The calorie reduction at this level is fifty percent. For a 200 lb. person, this will be 1,000 calories per day. By dividing this by six, it's 167 calories for each of the six meals. For this intensive plan,

1,000 calories will be burned by performing your six daily activities. The calories can be burned by using just one intensive activity along with the other five non-intensive activities. An alternative would be to burn the 1,000 calories with any combination of your six daily activities.

Consuming 1,000 calories and burning 1,000 calories a day leaves the 200 lb. person with a loss of 2,000 calories a day. The day of fasting will be for thirty-six hours, starting with your last meal of your sixth day then ending when you have your first meal on the first day of the new week. There will be no strenuous activities on this day. Fasting will be a loss of 2,000 calories. The loss for the week will be about 14,000 calories, which is four pounds. Eight weeks at this level will be about a thirty-two pound loss.

An example of a meal is one low calorie tortilla wrap, three ounces of turkey, one slice of tomato, and one teaspoon of mustard. This is about 164 calories, twenty-two grams of protein, five grams of fat, and twenty grams of carbohydrates. Create your own meals using similar calorie and nutritional content.

An example of a day's activities are two hours in the gym burning 600 calories, one hour outside riding a bicycle burning 300 calories, and a half hour of yoga burning 100 calories. For the non-intensive activities, for a half hour plant some flowers, spend an hour doing your favorite hobby, then go to a play for two hours. These are examples, use activities that are similar, producing the same results.

Extreme666 is the most challenging and rewarding Diet666 plan that you can configure. This is similar to the previous plan, just more intensive. The major difference is that you will be burning a significant number of calories on your day of fasting.

Be well prepared, at this level you will be pushing your limits. You must have a healthy mind and body to proceed. Be disciplined and consistent when proceeding with this plan. Consume nutritious meals with a high percentage of protein. Take a multivitamin and any necessary nutritional supplements. Because of the diminished daily calorie consumption, it can be challenging to get the proper amount of daily protein and other essential nutrients. You can do a few weeks at a variety of levels. For example, one week at low intensity, one week at medium intensity, one week at high intensity, then two weeks of extreme intensity. Create a plan that you are comfortable with. Choose the proper activities to burn the desired number of calories.

The daily calorie consumption will be at a sixty-five percent reduction. For a 200 lb. person, this will be a consumption of 700 total calories for each day. Each of the six meals will be 116 calories.

There will be activities chosen to burn 1,200 calories a day. On the day of fasting, activities will be used to burn 500 calories. When fasting, choose the amount of activities and the types of activities to lose the 500 calories. For the week, the weight loss will be 1,300 less per day from calorie restrictions. There will be 1,200 calories used by the activities. The fasting will be for thirty-six hours. It will be a loss of 2,000 calories from having no meals and 500 calories burned from performing activities. This will be a total loss of 2,500 calories from each of the six days, and the day of fasting you will also lose 2,500 calories. The total loss for the week will be 17,500 calories, or five pounds.

An example of a meal is a lettuce wrap made with leafy lettuce for the wrap, three ounces of turkey, and one tablespoon of diced sweet red pepper. This is 116 calories, eighteen grams of protein, three grams of fat, and five grams of carbohydrates. Use meals that are similar in calories and nutritional contents.

An example of a day's activities is two hours at the gym burning 600 calories, one hour doing an outdoor jog burning 300 calories, and a one-hour swim burning 300 calories. for the non-intensive activities, play an instrument for an hour, do a hobby for an hour, then play a video game for an hour. An example of the fasting day activities is one hour at the gym burning 300 calories and a one-hour outdoor walk burning 200 calories. When choosing activities, choose your own activities that will burn a similar amount of calories.

Maintenance Program

Congratulations, you have reached your goal! Now what? It's time to keep the weight off with a maintenance program. Keep in mind the variables of your water retention, this is most likely the result of salt consumption. If you increase your salt intake, your body will increase in weight from water retention. Avoid eating sugar and sugar products. Limit your complex carbohydrates. These foods can sharply increase your hunger besides adding unnecessary calories to your body. Be mindful of situations that might influence you to overeat and avoid them.

Try to have between three and six nutritious meals paced throughout the day. I recommend having at least three meals but six is best. Determine what your daily starting calorie count is. For a 180 lb. person, it's 180 x 10 for a total of 1,800 starting calories. If there are going to be three meals, they would be 600 calories each. If there are six meals, they would be 300 calories each.

Consider if during the day only a few calories are going to be burned by performing non-intensive activities, or if there are going to be intense workouts burning many calories. Calculate the calories used by activities into your plan. Do between three and six activities throughout the day, whether intensive or not. The day of fasting is no longer required but can be used as a maintenance tool when needed.

Choose a weight range that you want to stay in. If, for instance, your goal is to stay at 180 pounds, try to stay in the 175-180 pound range. If you go over 180 pounds, implement one of the Diet666 weight loss plans you have previously performed. Do this plan for a week then weigh yourself. Continue this weekly until you get yourself into your desired range again.

Another option is that after reaching your desired weight, stay on a very-low-intensity plan for a few weeks then slowly make the transition to the maintenance program. You will eventually find the right meal plan and activities to stay within your desired weight range.

Simplified Step-By-Step Guide

The following is a simplified guide to help you get started. Use this as a starting point. Change the intensity of the plan, the meals, and the activities as you see fit.

First, you must fully understand the entire book before starting. If you don't, it will be hard to create your ideal plan with the correct meals and activities. As you read the book, you will get a good feeling of how to proceed. Take notes and reread when necessary. Keeping a daily, weekly, and long-term journal will be helpful. Use a notebook to outline your personal Diet666 plan.

Step 1

Know what your ability is before you proceed. After fully understanding the concepts of Diet666, you will have an idea of the intensity that you want to start at. Discuss this with your medical doctor. I also recommend that you get a full examination and the full approval of your doctor.

Step 2

After being approved to proceed, work on your motivation. Set a realistic goal by considering your capabilities. Think hard and true about why you want to lose weight, be honest with yourself, then proceed with unstoppable determination. What keeps you motivated is important, you will think about this often during your weight loss journey.

Step 3

Determine the intensity of the plan that you're going to start with. Start with an intensity level that you can easily handle. If you start with something that's too intense for your capabilities, you will be at a disadvantage. You can intensify your plan on a daily or weekly basis. You can also reduce the intensity of your program if needed. Decide the timing of your activities, meals, the starting day, and your day of fasting, if applicable. Weigh yourself on the morning of your starting day. The first of your new week. You determine when your week starts.

Step 4

Choose meals that coincide with the intensity of your chosen diet plan. When choosing the contents of your meals, first determine the number of calories and amounts of protein, fat, and carbohydrates that are needed. If you choose to consume 1,200 calories for the day, you can have six 200-calorie meals that are high in protein, low in fat, and low in carbohydrates.

Step 5

Choose your activities in conjunction with the intensity level of your chosen plan. Create a list of activities you will be doing. Some of the activities can be work, personal responsibilities, everyday chores, hobbies, sports, the gym, etc.

Step 6

The day of fasting. This depends on the intensity level of your chosen plan. Determine when your fast starts and ends. Consume fewer than usual calories the day before your fasting day. Have the proper amount of sleep before starting your fast. Be prepared with a variety of liquids for your fast. Plan your day with low-intensity activities to help you get through the day. If you're doing Extreme666, your activities will be more intense. Keep a journal and adjust your plan as you see fit.

Chapter Six
How it Worked for Me

This chapter is the basics of how I configured my own personal plan, my journal, my personal experiences, and a few tips. I will cover my experiences from the very beginning to where I am now. Originally, I wanted to lose ten pounds at a rate of one pound a week. To my surprise, I accomplished this in one week. I surpassed my expectations by leaps and bounds. Using Diet666, I lost fifty-one pounds in seventeen weeks.

I will convey a little insight about myself so you will have a better understanding of my journey. I, Walter Labetti, sixty-three years of age, six-foot one-inch tall. I started Diet666 when I was 230 pounds. I am retired, presently living in Fort Lauderdale, Florida. I'm a retired NYC police officer that lived most of my life in Staten Island New York. Before moving to Florida, I lived in New Jersey for a while.

I've had many businesses including night clubs, restaurants, home improvements, and a security guard company to name a few. I have many hobbies including various types of art, music, watersports, skiing, motorcycle, and physical fitness in many forms. I have the freedom to schedule my activities with little restrictions. I have some basic knowledge of nutrition from being in the restaurant business. I configured menus and prepared meals.

The concept of Diet666 first started with my inspiration of learning how to surf. Originally, the surfing was to help me with my kiteboarding. Once I got into surfing, that was it, my life revolved around the surf. Except for one thing, it was very difficult for me to get up and ride a wave. I had a hard time popping up onto the board. My thought was, if I lost weight, surfing would be easier. I decided to lose a few pounds.

My motivation was based on the concept that if I lost some weight it would be easier for me to pop up onto the surfboard. I needed a solid, systematic weight loss plan. I didn't want to do what I have done many times. That is take the weight off then put it back on just as fast.

In my life I have tried many different types of diets. For instance, an all fish diet, an all meat diet, one daily meal diet, a counting calories diet, plus I was a vegetarian for ten years. I performed massive workouts, I tried an all liquid diet, I did the no fat diet, and of course, the no carbohydrate diets. I did some intense research into weight loss, eventually putting the pieces together.

I noticed there were some constants when comparing the weight loss methods, the ones that work and ones that don't. I noticed the flaws in some of the weight loss plans and others that are pure gimmicks. There is much more to a good weight loss program than just adjusting the food intake. It took some time for me to be confidant that I had the complete plan. I had to be sure that it wasn't just the typical, run-of-the-mill, quick-fix diet plan that you see on TV or read about in the tabloids.

Finally, I gave it a try. I was determined to lose ten pounds, one pound a week for ten weeks. After a few weeks of astonishing results, I decided to share this knowledge with everyone by writing this book. I believe that this Diet666 weight loss program can be used successfully, either short term for a few weeks or long term for months. Diet666 can be the way you live your life. That is, your long and rewarding life. This all-inclusive diet program was named Diet666 because of the basic concepts—six meals a day, six activities a day, six days a week, and a fast. Yes, it has that 666 mystical allure to it. Mysterious as it may be, until the concepts are fully understood.

My starting point was when I got fully motivated with a strong mindset, knowing that I'm going to do whatever it takes to lose the weight and be a better surfer. Prepared with the fundamentals of the Diet666 program, I set forth.

For no significant reason I started on a Tuesday morning. The first thing was to weigh myself and start a journal. My starting weight was 230 pounds. The next thing was to create a schedule. I took into consideration the timing of my activities and meals. This was easy because I have basically no mandatary, nonadjustable responsibilities. I found it easy to create my basic activity schedule then add the meals accordingly.

My week started on Tuesday, weighing myself in the morning. I consumed six meals plus performed six activities daily from Tuesday through Sunday, then I fasted on Monday. Technically, my fast started at the last meal that I had on Sunday then ended on my first meal that I had on Tuesday. My personal Diet666 plan was a variation of the medium-intensity level, the high-intensity level, and then the Extreme666 level.

As time went on, I had less calories for each meal and added more intensive workouts to my activity program. After reaching my desired weight, I switched to a maintenance program, which is where I am right now. I'm adjusting my gym workouts to gain muscle. I'm adding more protein and calories to my meals to support my muscle growth. I'm still adjusting my activities and meals so I can accomplish my goals. My maintenance program is low intensity without fasting. I want to stay in an area of 180 pounds and gain some muscle.

My Mental Outlook

If there is one thing that is going to get you to your goal weight it's your state of mind, considering you're healthy enough to carry out your chosen plan. For me, my weight is important because being too heavy makes my physical activities a lot harder. Less weight probably means I'll live a little longer, well, maybe! What better reason to lose weight? Perhaps looking better, feeling energetic, getting compliments, and having that great feeling of self-accomplishment. I so much looked forward to the experience of buying new cloths, like smaller sizes.

All along, every day, I looked forward to the day when I reached my goal weight. I was fired up with unstoppable determination. It just seems like every aspect of my life is better after losing all that weight. I noticed as I lost weight my determination increased. Seeing results is a strong driving force.

My Preference in Meals

To start with, I knew a little about nutrition but not enough to form a diet plan, so I did some in-depth research. I focused on the basics; protein, carbohydrates, and fat. My first meals were made from ingredients I was accustomed to. The first meals were sandwiches made with one slice of low calorie, high fiber bread, honey-maple turkey, and mustard. Eventually, I found wraps that are fifty calories made with whole wheat and flax seed. I use this wrap a lot. I add turkey or chicken and combine assorted vegetables for nutrition and diversity. Turkey wraps are my favorite. They are convenient, low in calories, and satisfying.

Other meals are beef jerky, broiled chicken breast, hard-boiled eggs, tuna, and other fish on occasion. I have protein drinks that are high in protein and not high in calories. When I go out for dinner, I avoid high carbohydrates and foods that are high in fat. I have high-protein meals. I drink mostly bottled sparkling water. I have my coffee with artificial sweetener and milk. I drink diet soda. I seldom drink alcoholic beverages.

I don't eat any types of pure sugar products, which is a primary rule. I limit my salt intake. Salt is generally unhealthy and also causes water retention. My consumption of carbohydrates is very limited. They have too many calories and will trigger hunger urges. My preferences when consuming complex carbohydrates are beans, nuts, and vegetables, and I seldom have fruit. I keep ripe, skinned bananas in the freezer for special occasions. They taste like ice cream. I avoid consuming fat, especially saturated fat, but having some healthy fat is necessary for a healthy diet.

When dieting at the Extreme666 intensity level, I will use lettuce wraps because of their lower calorie content. I take a daily multivitamin and a calcium supplement. When my diet is very low in fat, I take omega-3 fish oil supplements. When fasting, I drink water, orange flavored sparkling water, diet soda, tea, and coffee. It varies from time to time. Sometimes it's only water, other times it's a lot of tea. No sugar and little or no calories.

My Activity Preferences

My activities fall into two categories, either burning many calories or burning few calories. My activities are chosen for various purposes. Some activities are my personal responsibilities that must be done. For example, cleaning the pool, shopping, cooking, etc.

Some activities that I do are my various hobbies and there are many. Some of my hobbies are different types of art, playing the guitar or drums, reading, writing, gardening, ocean activities, motorcycle riding, etc. Some of these hobbies are intense but some are not. I go to the gym for two or more hours a day, six days a week, burning about 1,000 calories each time. I sometimes walk, run, or rollerblade outdoors, burning a significant number of calories.

I enjoy all my activities. There are some that burn more calories than others, but they all take up a time slot. My gym exercises are usually two hours or longer, doing aerobics on a treadmill, stair machine, or stationary bicycle, then an hour doing weight training. For each of my various weightlifting exercises, I use light weights and perform many repetitions. I use free weights or machines.

My six activities are basically a combination of my daily responsibilities, my hobbies, and the gym. I start with a simple activity plan for the day then adjust it as needed, sometimes things happen, and plans change.

My Way of Fasting

I choose to do my fasting on Mondays, for me it's a convenient day to do it. The actual time of fasting starts when I have my last meal on Sunday night then ends when I have my first meal on Tuesday. I always do more than a twenty-four-hour fast. It's more in the area of thirty-six hours. If my last meal is at nine p.m. on Sunday and my first meal is at nine a.m. on Tuesday, that's a thirty-six-hour fast. It's convenient for me to do it this way.

The day before my fast, I have fewer calories than usual and I avoid having salt. It seems that having fewer calories the day before the fast makes me less hungry during the fast. The body is adjusted to having fewer calories. I always get a good night's sleep, for me it's at least eight hours. When I wake up on Monday morning, I start my day with a cup coffee and take a multivitamin, a calcium supplement, and an omega-3 supplement. Throughout the day, I will be drinking bottled water, flavored sparkling water, tea, and coffee.

I plan my day with light activities. I will go shopping, go to a bookstore, go for a swim, or go for a walk on the beach. If I'm doing the fast at the Extreme666 level, I most likely will run outdoors to burn calories. At night, I might go to the movies, see a play, go to a concert, or a perhaps a sports event. At home I will read, write, play my guitar, or listen to music.

At the onset of hunger, I will have a caffeinated drink, hot or cold. Taking a shower or going for a swim eliminates hunger. I never get extremely hungry during the fast. I have done the fast for seventeen weeks in a row, every Monday. I never got to a point where I had to have food or any significant number of calories. The only calories I had was from milk in my coffee. Fasting is much easier than I thought. I always looked forward to the day of fasting, knowing that the next day I will be weighing myself and will be seeing the week's results.

Weighing Myself

I weigh myself when I wake up in the morning of the first day of my dieting week. For my plan, the starting day was always Tuesday, so every Tuesday morning when I got out of bed, unclothed, I weighed myself. I only weigh myself once a week and use that weight for my entire week's calorie calculations. Whatever the results are is perfectly fine, it all works out in the long run. Sometimes I lost more than expected and sometimes less.

My first week I lost twelve pounds. Most of the loss was due to me consuming very little amounts of salt. There were a couple of weeks when there was no weight loss even though I burned a massive amount of calories and was very restrictive with my calorie intake. After seventeen weeks I reached my goal. I lost fifty-one pounds, averaging three pounds a week. I found my Diet666 program exciting and I looked forward to the one time a week when I weighed myself.

During seventeen weeks of losing fifty-one pounds, I used the moderate, high intensity, and the Extreme666 intensity programs with some variations. Every Monday for seventeen weeks I did a full fast of about thirty-six hours. I will show you the weekly results of my seventeen-week journey.

My starting point was at a weight of 230 lbs.
Week 1, I lost 12 lbs., down to 218 lbs.
Week 2, I lost 3 lbs., down to 215 lbs.
Week 3, I lost zero pounds, remaining at 215 lbs.
Week 4, I lost 6 lbs., down to 209 lbs.
Week 5, I lost 2 lbs., down to 207 lbs.
Week 6, I lost 3 lbs., down to 204 lbs.
Week 7, I lost zero pounds, remaining at 204 lbs.
Week 8, I lost 4 lbs., down to 200 lbs.
Week 9, I lost 2 lbs., down to 198 lbs.
Week 10, I lost 3 lbs., down to 195 lbs.
Week 11, I lost 3 lbs., down to 198 lbs.
Week 12, I lost 2 lbs., down to 190 lbs.
Week 13, I lost 1 lb., down to 189 lbs.
Week 14, I lost 3 lbs., down to 186 lbs.
Week 15, I lost 3 lbs., down to 183 lbs.
Week 16, I lost zero pounds, remaining at 183 lbs.
Week 17, I lost 4 lbs., down to 179 lbs.

My First Week

During my first week, I lost twelve pounds even though according to my calculations, I should have lost four pounds. I contribute this to a loss of water weight because of my low salt consumption. The first day I weighed myself, I was 230 pounds. I multiply my weight by ten, giving me my starting negative calorie count of 2,300, which I will use every day for this current week. The next week I will weigh myself and this number will change for that week. The 2,300 negative starting calories represents the number of calories I will use for the day to exist. This means if I didn't burn any extra calories and I didn't consume any calories I would have lost 2,300 calories at the end of the day.

When I fasted that week, I lose the 2,300 calories plus 100 calories from minor activities for a total loss of 2,400 calories. I don't count small amounts of calories, such as the milk in my coffee, nor do I count small amounts of calories burned, such as driving short distances. For me, it gets too complicated to count every single calorie.

<u>Day one</u>

I started my day with a cup of coffee, which I do every day.
Activity 1, at 10 a.m. I was at the gym for 2 hrs., burning 700 calories.
Activity 2, at 12 p.m. I walked for 5 miles, burning 500 calories.
Meal 1, at 1 p.m. I had a small mango, 100 calories.
Meal 2, at 4 p.m. I had a turkey sandwich, 200 calories.
Activity 3, at 4:10 p.m. I cooked dinner for 1hr., burning 100 calories.
Activity 4, at 5:10 p.m. I cleaned my pool for 1/2 hr., burning 100 calories.
Meal 3, at 6 p.m. I had a salad of tuna, chickpeas, and tomato, 500 calories.
Activity 5, at 7 p.m. I read a book for 1 hr., zero calories.
Activity 6, at 8 p.m. I played the guitar for 1/2 hr., zero calories.
Meal 4, at 9 p.m. I had two slices of cheese, 200 calories.
Meal 5, at 10 p.m. I had a banana, 100 calories.
Meal 6, at 11 p.m. I had walnuts, 300 calories.

The results: I started with a negative calorie count of 2,300 plus 100 calories I used from my minor activities and another 1,400 calories I burned by performing my six activities. This is a total of 3,800 negative calories. I consumed 1,400 calories from my six meals, leaving me with a total loss of 2,400 calories for the day.

<u>Day two</u>

Activity 1, at 12 p.m. I went rollerblading for 1 hr., burning 400 calories.
Meal 1, at 4 p.m. I had a turkey sandwich, 400 calories.
Activity 2, at 4:30 p.m. I went swimming for 1/2 hr., burning 100 calories.
Activity 3, at 6 p.m. I prepared food for a party for 1/2 hr., burning zero calories.
Activity 4, at 8 p.m. I was at a party for 3 hrs., burning 100 calories.
Meal 2, at 8:30 p.m. I had a salad, 600 calories.
Meal 3, at 9:30 p.m. I had a hotdog, 300 calories.
Meal 4, at 10:30 p.m. I had a banana, 100 calories.
Meal 5, at 11 p.m. I had mixed nuts, 200 calories.
Activity 5, at 11:15 p.m., I read a book for a 1/2 hr., zero calories.
Activity 6, at 11:45 p.m. I played the guitar for 1/2 hr., zero calories.
Meal 6, at 12:15 a.m. I had two slices of cheese, 200 calories.

The results: A starting negative calorie count of 2,300 plus 100 calories used by my minor activities and another 600 calories used by my six activities. I consumed 1,800 calories from my six meals, leaving me with a loss of 1,200 calories.

<u>Day three</u>

Meal 1, at 11 a.m. I had a turkey sandwich, 100 calories.
Activity 1, at 12 p.m. I was at the gym for 2 hrs., burning 700 calories.
Activity 2, at 2:30 p.m. I went shopping for 1 hr., burning 100 calories.
Activity 3, at 4 p.m. I planted a tree in my back yard, which took an hour, burning 200 calories.
Meal 2, at 5 p.m. I had a hard-boiled egg, 100 calories.

Meal 3, at 6 p.m. I had a few pieces of assorted cheese, 200 calories.
Meal 4, at 7 p.m. I had cabbage and bean soup, 500 calories.
Activity 4, at 7:30 p.m. I read a book for 1 hr., zero calories.
Activity 5, at 9 p.m. I played the guitar for 1/2 hr., zero calories.
Meal 5, at 9:30 p.m. I had hazelnuts, 100 calories.
Meal 6, at 10 p.m. I had an eggplant parmesan sandwich, 600 calories.
Activity 6, at 11 p.m. I was writing for an hour, zero calories.

The results: A starting negative calorie count of 2,300 plus 100 calories used by my minor activities and another 1,000 calories used by my six activities. I consumed 1,600 calories from six meals, leaving me with a loss of 1,700 calories.

Day four

Meal 1, at 11 a.m. I had a turkey sandwich, 100 calories.
Activity 1, at 1:30 p.m. I walked for 2 hrs., burning 500 calories.
Meal 2, at 4 p.m. I had a turkey sandwich, 100 calories.
Activity 2, at 4:30 p.m. I cleaned my back yard for 1/2 hr., zero calories.
Activity 3, at 5 p.m. I swam for 1/2 hr., burning 100 calories.
Meal 3, at 5:30 p.m. I had tuna and arugula salad, 200 calories.
Activity 4, at 6 p.m. I cleaned my garage for 1/2 hr., zero calories.
Activity 5, at 6:30 p.m. I played the drums for 1/2 hr., burning 100 calories.
Meal 4, at 7 p.m. I had a turkey sandwich, 100 calories.
Activity 6, at 8 p.m. I read a book for 1/2 hr., zero calories.
Meal 5, at 8:30 p.m. I had macadamia nuts, 100 calories.
Meal 6, at 10 p.m. I had an eggplant parmesan sandwich, 600 calories.

The results: A starting negative calorie count of 2,300 plus 100 calories used by my minor activities and another 700 calories used by my six activities. I consumed 1,200 calories from my six meals, leaving me with a loss of 1,900 calories.

<u>Day five</u>

Meal 1, at 10 a.m. I had a turkey sandwich, 100 calories.
Activity 1, at 12 p.m. I was at the gym for 2 hrs., burning 700 calories.
Activity 2, at 3 p.m. I cleaned my back yard for 1/2 hr., zero calories.
Activity 3, at 4:30 p.m. I cooked dinner for 1/2 hr., zero calories.
Meal 2, at 5 p.m. I had an arugula and cheese salad, 200 calories.
Activity 4, at 6 p.m. I read a book for 1/2 hr., zero calories.
Meal 3, at 6:30 p.m. I had a turkey sandwich, 100 calories.
Meal 4, at 7 p.m. I had hazelnuts, 100 calories.
Activity 5, at 7:30 p.m. I played my guitar for 1/2 hr., zero calories.
Meal 5, at 8 p.m. I ate a banana, 100 calories.
Activity 6, at 9 p.m. I read a book for an hour, zero calories.
Meal 6, at 10 p.m. I had beef jerky, 300 calories.

The results: A starting negative calorie count of 2,300 plus 100 calories used by my minor activities and another 700 calories used by my six activities. I consumed 900 calories from my six meals, leaving me with a loss of 2,200 calories.

<u>Day six</u>

Meal 1, at 9 a.m. I had a banana, 100 calories.
Activity 1, at 12 p.m. I walked for 2 hrs., burning 500 calories.
Activity 2, at 3 p.m. I went shopping for 1/2 hr., zero calories.
Meal 2, at 5 p.m. I had tuna and arugula salad, 200 calories.
Activity 3, at 6 p.m. I swam for 1/2 hr., burning 100 calories.
Activity 4, at 7 p.m. I read a book for 1/2 hr., zero calories.
Meal 3, at 7:30 p.m. I had a hard-boiled egg, 100 calories.
Meal 4, at 9 p.m. I had pistachio nuts, 400 calories.
Activity 5, at 9:30 p.m. I played my guitar for 1/2 hr., zero calories.
Meal 5, at 10 p.m. I had a turkey sandwich, 100 calories.
Activity 6, at 10:30 p.m. I read a book for 1 hr., zero calories.
Meal 6, at 11:30 p.m. I ate a banana, 100 calories.

The results: A starting negative calorie count of 2,300 plus 100 calories used by my minor activities and another 600 calories used by my six activities. I consumed 1,000 calories from my six meals, leaving me with a loss of 2,000 calories.

<u>Day seven, the fast</u>

The results: A starting negative calorie count of 2,300 plus 100 calories used by my minor activities. This was a total loss of 2.400 calories for the day.

The total number of calories I lost for the week was 13,800 calories.

My Rewards

For me, the best benefit is for me to have full control of my weight. This in itself is an amazing accomplishment, a great feeling for sure. Having lost the weight and by knowing all the principles in this book, I will always be able to keep my weight in check. There's a great feeling of self-accomplishment and self-control, not only by losing the weight, but also by organizing my daily activities.

The concepts that are presented in this book gave me the insight into nutrition and exercise. Diet666 also showed me a path toward living a healthy and productive life. My ability to focus on my hobbies and interests drastically increased, and I developed a strong type of discipline. It's nice to look in the mirror and see myself in a different light, like seeing some muscle and not fat. Breathing better and running faster and longer are also great gifts.

After losing the weight, I feel lighter on my feet and anything physical is much easier. It finally got easier for me to pop up onto my surfboard and my swimming ability increased. Hopefully, my kiteboarding and skiing ability will increase; I didn't try them yet. Riding my motorcycle is more comfortable. It was a pleasure buying new clothes. I went from a tight size thirty-eight pants to a comfortable size thirty-four. My shirts went from a size XXL to a large. The size thirty-eight pants and the XXL shirts were all given away, never to be seen again.

Some people say, "You lost too much weight!" How I love it! I kind of feel like I did when I was a teenager with all that energy and enthusiasm. I could never have imagined that I would wind up being the same weight that I was in my early twenties. I'm still amazed. I can definitely say that being overweight slowed me down, but not anymore! Last but not least, perhaps Diet666 will keep me alive a little longer. Hopefully you, also.

My Future Expectations

Now after losing the weight, I have decided to build some muscle mass. I did lose some muscle along the way. I plan on intensifying my weightlifting exercises by using heavier than usual weights and also intensifying the exercises I do with the machines. I will still do a moderate aerobics program to stay fit.

I must also add the right amount of protein and calories to support my muscle growth. If I gain a moderate amount of weight that is not proportionate to my muscle mass, I will choose a maintenance program to lose the unnecessary fat. This may go back and forth a few times until I get it right. I will focus on getting the right balance of muscle mass, the proper activities, protein consumption, and the correct number of calories. I plan on having more diverse meals while maintaining the proper nutrition and also having the right number of calories. I want Diet666 to become a way of life, to do it like clockwork with little conscious effort.

A Few Tips

The very first thing to do is acquire the necessary motivation. Search your soul to find every reason why you want to lose weight. There will be that one magic reason that will be your driving force. This will give you that unstoppable determination, ensuring your success. For me, it was to help me be a better surfer.

Ensure that you are physically and mentally fit for the intensity of the program you intend to use.

In the beginning, create a program that you can easily handle. If your usual, daily calorie consumption is 4,000 calories, don't start with a drastically reduced calorie consumption of 600 calories. First, focus on the timing of your meals and activities then limit your calories and add more intensive activities.

Are you in a hurry? Fifty pounds can be lost in the course of a year by losing one pound a week, or you can lose the fifty pounds in twenty-five weeks by losing two pounds a week. You can lose fifty-one pounds in seventeen weeks by losing three pounds a week.

Create a program that you can handle. As time goes on, adjust your personal Diet666 program as needed. It's all right to do an intense program one week then a less intensive one the following week.

Sugar and sugar products are to be avoided at all costs. Besides the unnecessary calories, sugar makes you hungry.

While I'm limiting my calories drastically, my nutrition becomes deficient in some areas. I take a multivitamin, a calcium supplement, and an omega-3 fish oil supplement.

It's important to lose some weight every day, even if it's a little. This keeps the body trained at using body fat for energy. This process helps keep hunger away.

After a few weeks I started to use low-calorie wraps or lettuce wraps, which are very low in calories. I found this better than consuming sandwiches.

Get the proper amount of sleep, for me it's between eight and ten hours. If you are sleep deficient your body can interpret this for hunger.

Stay hydrated. If you're not properly hydrated your body can also interpret this for hunger.

Water retention can account for a significant amount of weight. This can be controlled by reducing your salt intake. After limiting your salt intake and losing that water weight, remember that this weight will come right back if a large amount of salt is consumed.

My tip for fasting is to not consume a lot of calories the previous day and think this will get you through the next day. To the contrary, this will influence you to be hungry. Eat fewer calories than you're accustomed to. Fasting was a lot easier than I thought it would be.

Tips For When You Stray From Your Diet Plan

An ice-cold shower will instantly destroy hunger. Catch yourself before your hunger reaches critical mass. Consume a large amount of protein and fat if necessary, with no or little carbohydrates. Protein from meat, poultry, or fish is best for this purpose. Have one, two, or three caffeinated zero-calorie drinks. Perform an activity that is intensive or mind focusing. Both work well. Go for a run, a brisk walk, a swim, or take a cold shower.

If all else fails, and you consumed more than desired calories, don't try to get even in one day. Stick to your basic plan, be confident, it will all work out in the long run. Analyze the situation. What caused this event? Could it have been caused by a social situation, feeling compelled to eat? Perhaps you had too many carbohydrates and not enough protein. Were you deficient in sleep, liquids, or activities? Did you workout too hard and get fatigued? Correct the problem. From my experience, being sick, fatigued, or having a minor injury can cause me to be overly hungry. I balance this out with a few naps throughout the day and follow through with a less intensive diet plan.

At social functions it can be compelling to overeat and drink. This can be overcome with the proper planning of meals and activities. Socialize with words, not with high calorie food and alcoholic drinks. Avoid alcohol, it will impair your good judgement. Be patient. It seems like we all want the fat to come off our hips first. Unfortunately, at least for me, the fat came off my hips last. Happily, it did happen. Ironically, when I had the least amount of hunger is when I was consuming fewer than 1,000 calories and burning 1,500 calories a day.

For my vegan friends I suggest creating meals with complete proteins that include healthy fats while avoiding high amounts of carbohydrates.

Diet666 would be fun to do with friends, family members, or groups of like-minded people. Creating meals together, doing activities of mutual interest together, and sharing the day fasting can be rewarding. It would be nice to have a support group.

Maintaining a Journal

For a daily journal, put your meals and activities in chronological order. Include the meal's contents along with their calories. Include the activities and any calories that are burned. At the end of each day, calculate the number of calories you lost. Each week calculate the estimated calories that you lost and compare that to the weight you are now, when you weigh yourself.

The following are pages for your personal notes and journals.

<u>The health log</u> can be used to record your before and after health status, your starting weight, blood pressure, cholesterol, etc. Also make notes of any concerns, conditions, or improvements.

<u>Health Log</u>

The motivation page can be used to write down all the reasons why you are determined to lose weight. Why will I succeed? Why will I not give up? Reflect on this page from time to time.

<u>Notes for your goals</u> can be used for the weight loss you want to achieve and other goals that you may want to accomplish while doing your Diet666 program, such as education, hobbies, music, sports, muscle building etc.

<u>The helpful calorie calculations page</u> can be used to let you know how many calories you lost during the day. First by determining your starting negative calorie count, then by determining how many calories were used during the day, and finally the number of calories that you consumed during the day.

For example, your weight is 270 lbs. x 10 = 2,700 calories. Add the 100 calories used from minor activities, add the calories used from your daily activities, say for instance 700 calories, this would be a negative calorie count of 3,500 calories. Now subtract the calories you consumed from your six meals, say for instance 1,500 calories, this would be a total loss of 2,000 calories for the day.

<u>Calorie Calculations</u>

Your weight ________   x 10   =   ____________

add the calories burned from minor activities   <u>100</u>

add the calories burned from your activities   __________

Total all the above calories   =   __________

Subtract the calories you had from your six meals   __________

This is the total calories lost for the day   __________

<u>Notes for meals</u> is where you can jot down what meals work for you, what needs to be adjusted, and whatever you think is significant pertaining to nutrition and calories.

<u>Notes for Meals</u>

<u>Notes for activities</u> is where you can take notes about what activities are good for you, what works to burn fat, and what keeps you away from hunger. Whatever you think is necessary.

<u>Notes for fasting</u> is where you can take notes about what you can do to make your fast pleasurable, what activities and drinks to use, and how to handle your hunger. What works and what doesn't.

Responsibility notes is where you can list your daily responsibilities. These are the things you must do, and you have to plan your Diet666 program around. List the things you can and can't reschedule or eliminate.

<u>Scheduling notes</u> is where you outline a preliminary or set schedule. Consider your responsibilities, pick a convenient day to fast, and also the times of your meals and activities.

<u>Scheduling Notes</u>

The daily journal is where you create your schedule for the day. Set the times for your meals and activities. Use this for one or many days. Alter it as you see fit. You can us this for what you plan, for what you have accomplished, or both. Consider your personal responsibilities. A pencil or erasable pen might be best for this section.

<u>Daily Journal</u>

<u>The weekly journal</u> is where you record the results of each day. Either simply record your daily weight loss or be very thorough including every meal and activity. The times, the number of calories for each meal, and the calories used during each activity. It's your choice.

<u>Weekly Journal</u>

This is the start of your new way of life. This is the beginning, use this book to control your weight and also control your way of living. The best of luck to you, share your experience with your friends. Spread the word, perhaps you will change someone's life for the best.

Thanks for being part of the Diet666 community. Good luck!

Walter Labetti

Diet666.com